HIT
RESET

HIT RESET

REVOLUTIONARY YOGA
FOR ATHLETES

ERIN TAYLOR

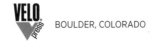 BOULDER, COLORADO

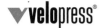 velopress®

3002 Sterling Circle, Suite 100
Boulder, Colorado 80301-2338 USA
(303) 440-0601 · Fax (303) 444-6788 · E-mail velopress@competitorgroup.com

Distributed in the United States and Canada by Ingram Publisher Services

A Cataloging-in-Publication record for this book is available from the Library of Congress.
ISBN 978-1-937715-42-7

For information on purchasing VeloPress books, please call (800) 811-4210, ext. 2138, or visit www.velopress.com.

This paper meets the requirements of ANSI/NISO Z39.48-1992 (Permanence of Paper).

Art direction by Vicki Hopewell
Interior design by Samira Selod and Vicki Hopewell

Photography by Justin Bailie, cover, pp. 4–5, 9–15, 17, 31–33, 37–46, 47 (top), 48–53, 55–56, 60, 63–65, 72–75, 77–83, 86, 98–103, 106–107, 109, 111–115, 117–119, 122–138, 142–143, 146–147, 149–156, 158–161, 163, 165–169, 196, 197 (left and middle), 200; Hilary Dahl, p. viii; James Finlay, pp. 29, 47 (bottom), 85, 140–141, 195; Nils Nilsen, p. 171; and Claire Pepper, pp. 18–19, 22–28, 57, 66–69, 70, 87, 90, 92–95, 97, 105, 197 (right), 199; photo retouching by Paula Gillen and Elizabeth Riley

Women's apparel (except Linsey Corbin) provided by Oiselle; yoga equipment provided by Manduka; locations courtesy of Green Lake Community Center, High Desert Crossfit, Mountain View High School, University of Washington, and ZUM Fitness

16   17   18 / 10   9   8   7   6   5   4   3   2   1

To you, the athletes
of the Reset Revolution

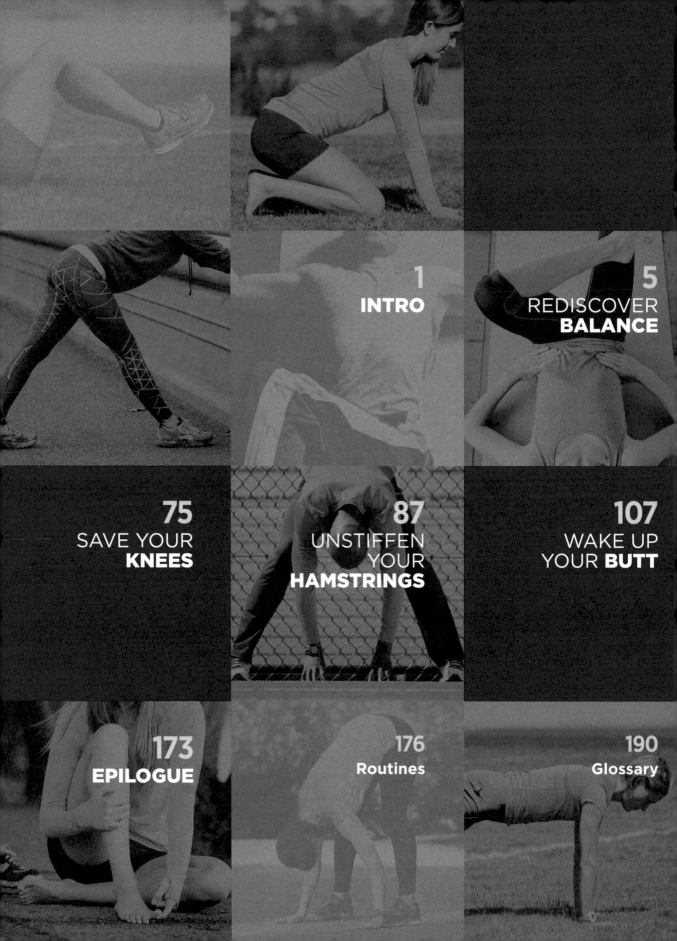

1 INTRO

5 REDISCOVER BALANCE

75 SAVE YOUR KNEES

87 UNSTIFFEN YOUR HAMSTRINGS

107 WAKE UP YOUR BUTT

173 EPILOGUE

176 Routines

190 Glossary

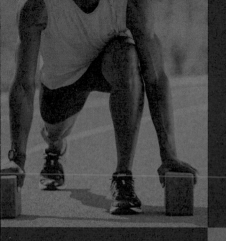

19
BREATHE &
FOCUS

33
STRENGTHEN
YOUR **CORE**

57
BALANCE
YOUR
FOUNDATION

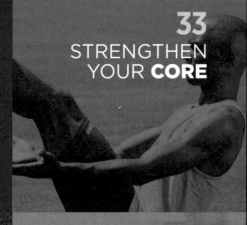

119
MOBILIZE &
STABILIZE
YOUR **HIPS**

143
SORT OUT
YOUR
SHOULDERS

161
UNSTICK
YOUR
SIDE BODY

194
Acknowledgments

196
About the
Athletes

199
About the
Author

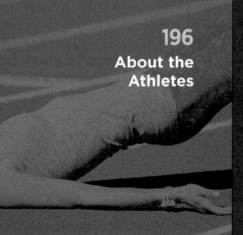

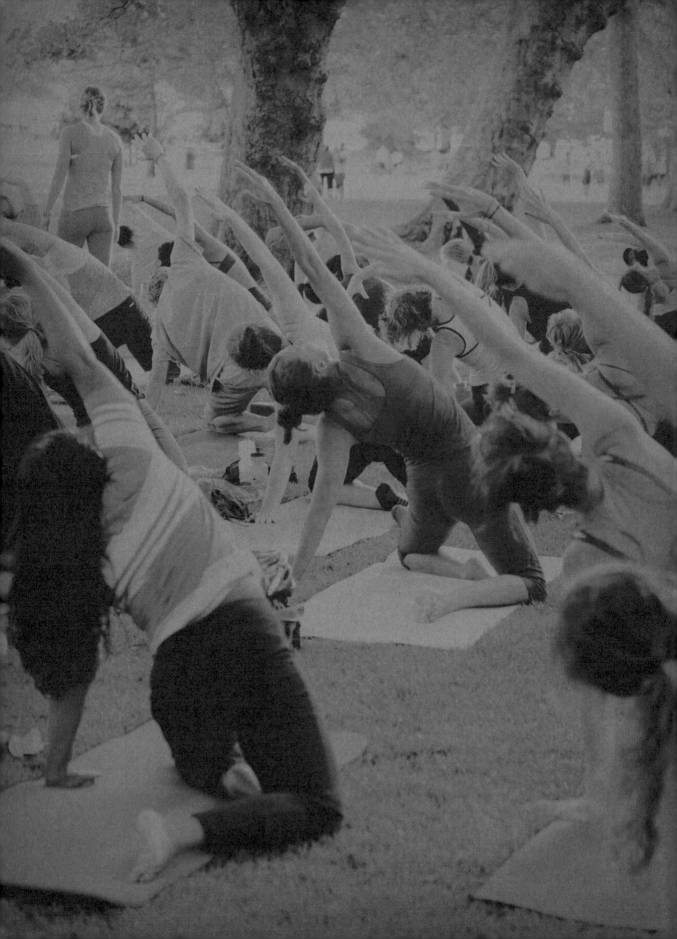

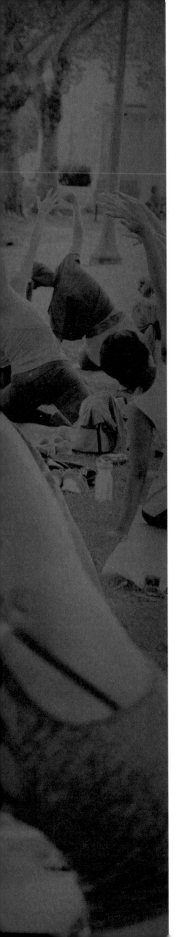

INTRO

ATHLETE FIRST, YOGI SECOND

I was a reluctant yogi. I still don't often use that word to describe myself.

As a collegiate basketball player, I thought yoga was boring at first, time that could be better spent on the court or in the weight room. It wasn't until I was sidelined by a spinal injury from overtraining that I got real about what was going on in my body—that I wasn't impressing anyone with my pain threshold, least of all myself.

Yoga was the Reset that helped me bring things back into balance, and although no sport-specific yoga solutions existed at that time, I quickly realized that when used in a relevant way, yoga equals balance, and balance equals winning.

RESET = A yoga solution that eases imbalance

FOR ATHLETES, INJURIES ARE DEVASTATING

There's nothing more disheartening than busting your ass to reach your peak only to end up injured and robbed of your chance to achieve your goals. After feeling the burn of a season spent on the sidelines, I knew more athletes would benefit from yoga's balance-inducing superpowers.

When I set out post-college to help athletes, the "yoga for athletes" space was a bit of an abyss, which forced me to think critically about what I was practicing and teaching and, more important, why. Athletes have been told that yoga will make them better at their sports, but the dots have to be connected. It's not just about doing yoga—it's how you do it. Certain poses might look cool on social media, but being able to put your foot behind your head isn't going to help you run faster or jump higher.

Over the last decade, I've dedicated myself to finding yoga's solutions to real problems and helping as many people as possible avoid the pain of imbalance—stress, injuries, and illness. These functional practices are practical, regardless of your sport or favorite fitness endeavor, whether you're a recreational or elite athlete or simply focused on better health and fitness. You can Hit Reset to become stronger and more resilient in as little as five minutes a day.

BALANCE IS A GAME CHANGER

Throughout this book you'll find practical tools to help you Hit Reset:

- **Problems and Solutions:** Understand how your body is designed to work.

- **Self-Test and Correct:** Become more aware of your unique imbalances and how to ease them.

- **Hit Reset:** Do the routines to bring things back into balance.

- **Game Plan:** Think about what you're doing and why.

HIT RESET SOLVES PROBLEMS

Organized by different areas of the body, this book presents straightforward explanations of some of the most common problems—imbalances—athletes suffer from today. Simple self-tests followed by practical, prescriptive solutions help you assess and correct issues that if left unchecked are likely to leave you injured and limit your potential. I've also included FAQs and techniques to make yoga more accessible and effective for you. It's my hope that you will use the knowledge and inspiration in this book to do yoga in a way that directly supports your unique and ambitious goals.

You'll feel more easeful when you rediscover balance and find a way to sustain it within your active lifestyle. You'll realize that while things aren't always easy, they don't have to be quite so hard. Accomplish this, and you will close the gap between where you are now and where you want to be.

WELCOME TO THE
RESET REVOLUTION

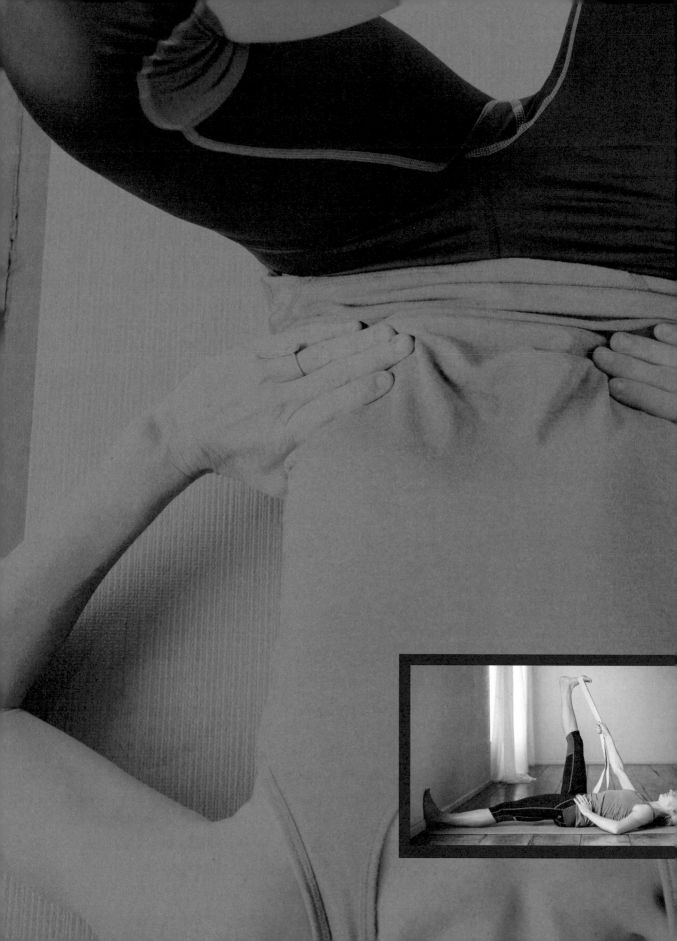

REDISCOVER
BALANCE

You are engineered for balance, so it makes sense that you're at your best when you're in balance.

Sustaining equilibrium between left and right, top and bottom, front and back—as well as work and rest—will help protect you from injuries, boost your performance, and optimize your fitness of any kind. Balance helps close the performance gap—it maximizes your potential.

Ultimately, it's up to each of us to continually redefine balance at the intersection of strength and flexibility, between effort and ease, in a way that supports us in achieving our unique goals.

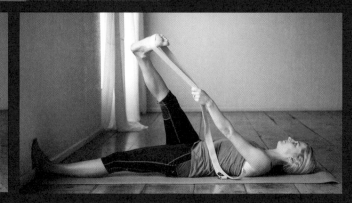

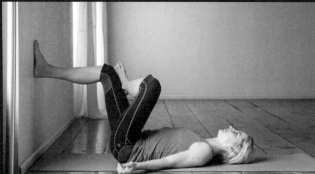

The imbalance problem

The reality is that wear and tear from working out and playing the sports you love, coupled with life's heavy workloads, can easily leave you underperforming, injured, or just plain burned out. In sports and in life, balance has become more elusive—and endeavoring to find your way back to it has become revolutionary. Ironically, our most natural state—balance—has become a radical ideal.

Here's the thing: Your body is a highly intelligent, integrated unit. Your biomechanics—the way your bones, connective tissue, and muscles are engineered to work together—are optimized when your body is balanced, but your body will do all kinds of less-than-ideal things in response to imbalance in order to keep you going.

Imbalance ultimately results in compensation, which is every athlete's worst enemy. If you fail to become aware of your imbalances and address them in a systematic way, your body will compensate—do whatever is necessary to keep you moving—and injury is inevitable. Be honest … that will suck. Consider the law of compensation: When your movement meets restriction and you continue to apply force, that force will transfer to the next available point of least resistance. If you force yourself through pain in one area, you'll inevitably cause pain in another area as well.

IMBALANCE → COMPENSATION → **INJURY**

Compensation =
The body's intrinsic and subconscious effort
to find balance
in the presence of dysfunction

Balance = Equilibrium

SOLUTION
THE **YOGA SOLUTION**

You have to earn balance, and yoga is a viable solution. Yoga equips you with insights into your imbalances and resulting compensation patterns, and gives you skills to systematically correct yourself back to a happy medium. But for yoga to work, you have to be real about where you are and take consistent action—you have to be aware of your imbalances and willing to respond accordingly day to day and moment to moment—otherwise you'll simply spend your time on the mat reinforcing your existing problems.

Everyone says to listen to your body, yet few take the time to respond. It's hard to fit one more thing into our busy schedules; it's true. But ironically, it's the times when we're too busy that we are most in need of some correction and benefit the most from slowing down and checking in with ourselves. Spending five minutes a day addressing a specific imbalance is more effective than attending one yoga class a week. Whether you have a few minutes or an hour to spend, approach your time on your mat as a real break—a Reset—rather than another addition to your to-do list.

USE YOGA TO SUSTAIN BALANCE

HIT RESET
TO REDISCOVER BALANCE

ROUTINE

✔ **Establish a Blueprint for Center** (p. 9)

BENEFITS

> Reestablish neutral alignment

> Assess your compensation patterns

PRACTICE	Post-workout/recovery
HOW LONG	Hold for 5–10 breaths per pose
PROPS	Strap, belt, or tie
RED FLAGS	Spinal compensation via back bending or side bending Knee discomfort

> *Most people have a body structure that is pretty symmetric, and the right-to-left imbalances they have aren't from bones, but rather how they control their bones. The quality of motion you have can be improved and refined. Take time to identify your imbalances, and take direction to bring your body back to symmetry. It's one of the best uses of your time as an athlete to ensure you reach your goals and hit a new PR."* —JAY DICHARRY, PHYSICAL THERAPIST AND RESEARCHER

FRAZZLED IS NOT FIT

ESTABLISH A BLUEPRINT FOR **CENTER**

Use this routine post-workout or on rest days to reestablish a sense of center, and practice maneuvering from there. Lying down with your feet on the wall mimics standing and gives you the opportunity to observe (without the work of standing and balancing) how your body compensates as you start moving your legs around, yielding powerful insights into your imbalances.

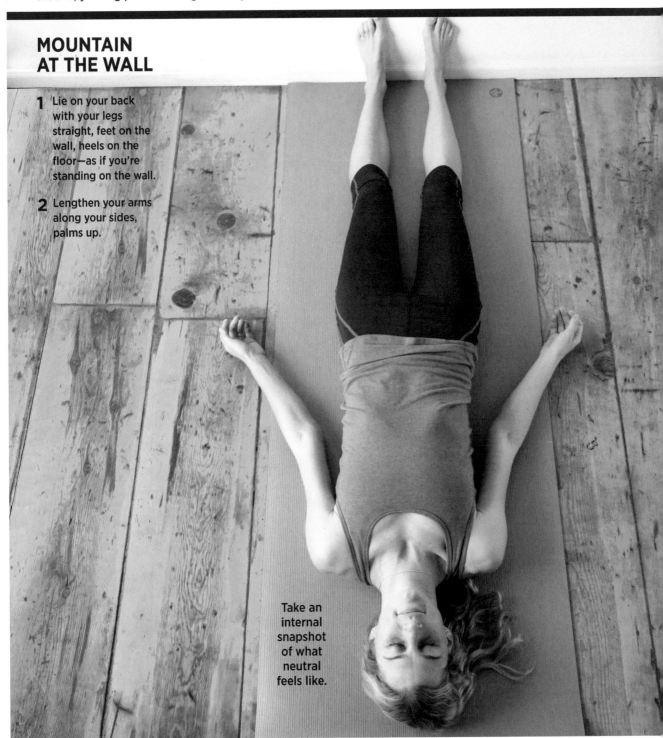

MOUNTAIN AT THE WALL

1 Lie on your back with your legs straight, feet on the wall, heels on the floor—as if you're standing on the wall.

2 Lengthen your arms along your sides, palms up.

Take an internal snapshot of what neutral feels like.

FIGURE 4
AT THE WALL

1 Lie on your back and put your feet flat on the wall so that your knees are bent at about a 90-degree angle—if your back feels uncomfortable, move farther away from the wall.

2 Cross one ankle over your other knee, keeping that foot flexed.

3 Bring your hands onto your waist to feel if the space between your ribs and hips is even on your right and left sides. If needed, slide your foot farther up the wall or move away from the wall to neutralize your spine.

Repeat on your other side.

>> Resist the urge to push your crossed leg forward with your hands—it forces your spine out of neutral and does nothing to deepen the stretch.

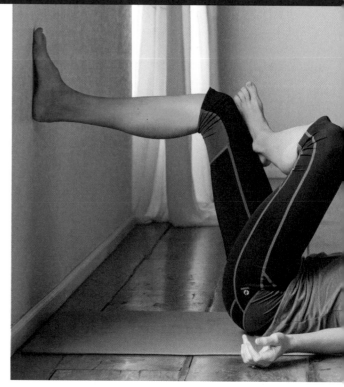

FAQ What am I really feeling?

As an athlete, you're well-versed in going hard and fast. But when you roll out your mat, it's important to slow down enough that you can more consciously discern what's going on in your body. If you go too hard, too fast, you'll miss out on valuable insights and your muscles are more likely to fight you, which is super-counterproductive and increases injury risk.

Consider the fact that sensations can be deceiving. Whether engaging or stretching a muscle, when you place an unfamiliar demand on that muscle, you're likely to experience some discomfort. The key is to clearly distinguish between the discomfort of improvement (good!) and the discomfort of injury (bad!). For example, after asking your hamstrings to engage and shorten to support your forward motion on your run, if you ask them to work toward the opposite extreme— stretch and lengthen when you reach for your toes post-workout—it might not feel great. A dull, general aching sensation in the muscle belly—the middle, meatiest part—is common and should be embraced, whereas sharper, more acute sensations in specific spots closer to joints should serve as red flags. Feel for your edge—a strong sensation that isn't painful. When you are unsure where

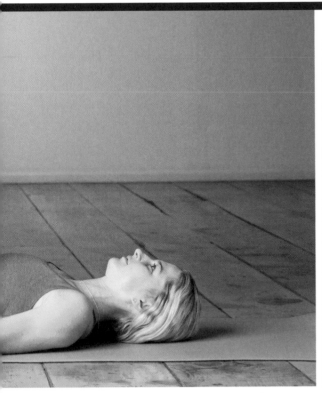

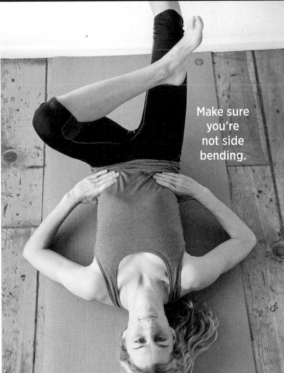

Make sure you're not side bending.

exactly the stretch is happening, engage the muscle, which will draw in more blood flow and reorient you to the muscle belly. When stretching safely, this is where you will feel the most sensation.

While pushing through pain might be familiar to you, that approach won't serve you when it comes to finding balance. Find your stopping point and stop there. And always resist the urge to compare yourself to others. Instead, be honest about where you are right now. Ask yourself, what am I really feeling?

After all, how pissed off would you be if you injured yourself doing yoga? Exactly.

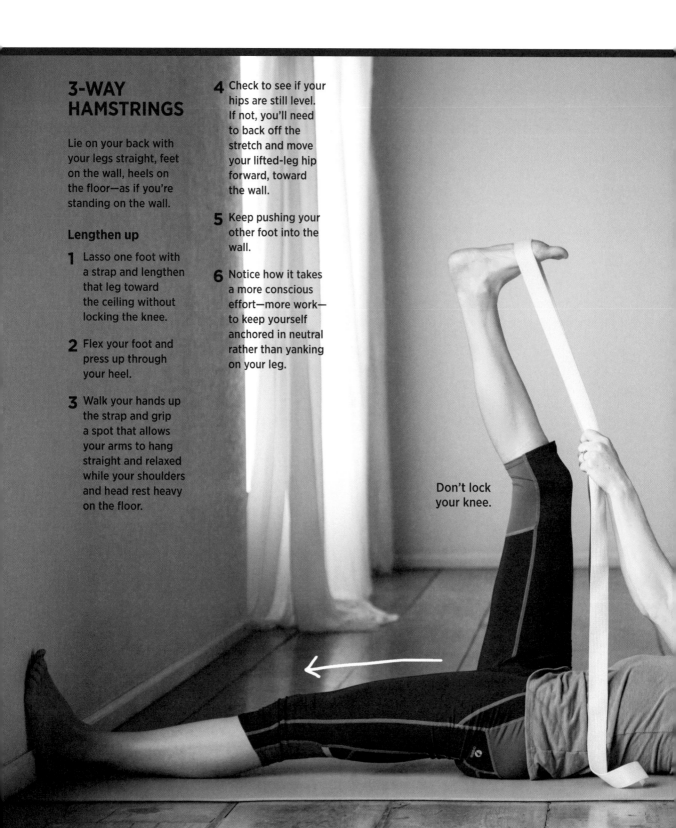

3-WAY HAMSTRINGS

Lie on your back with your legs straight, feet on the wall, heels on the floor—as if you're standing on the wall.

Lengthen up

1 Lasso one foot with a strap and lengthen that leg toward the ceiling without locking the knee.

2 Flex your foot and press up through your heel.

3 Walk your hands up the strap and grip a spot that allows your arms to hang straight and relaxed while your shoulders and head rest heavy on the floor.

4 Check to see if your hips are still level. If not, you'll need to back off the stretch and move your lifted-leg hip forward, toward the wall.

5 Keep pushing your other foot into the wall.

6 Notice how it takes a more conscious effort—more work— to keep yourself anchored in neutral rather than yanking on your leg.

Don't lock your knee.

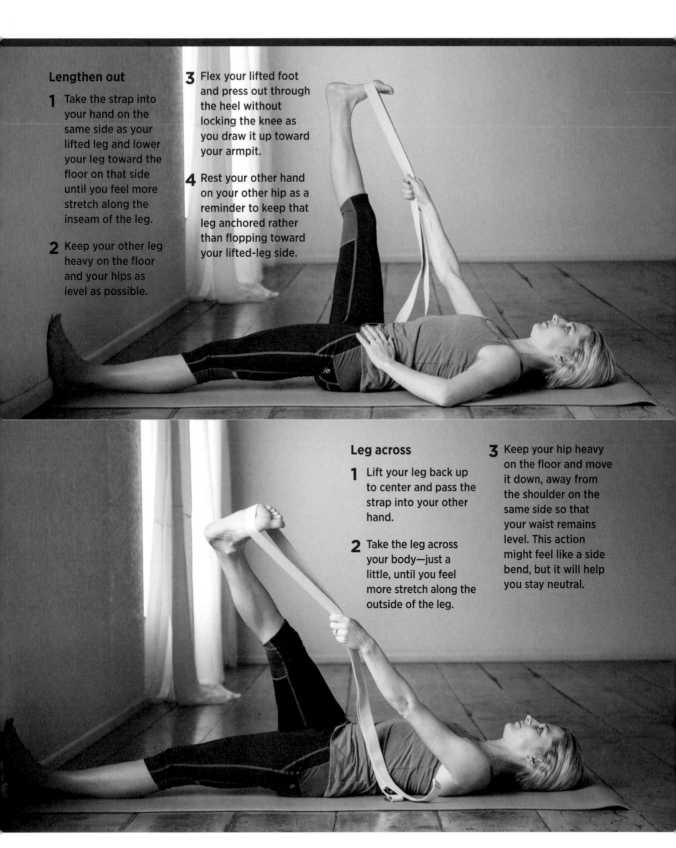

Lengthen out

1 Take the strap into your hand on the same side as your lifted leg and lower your leg toward the floor on that side until you feel more stretch along the inseam of the leg.

2 Keep your other leg heavy on the floor and your hips as level as possible.

3 Flex your lifted foot and press out through the heel without locking the knee as you draw it up toward your armpit.

4 Rest your other hand on your other hip as a reminder to keep that leg anchored rather than flopping toward your lifted-leg side.

Leg across

1 Lift your leg back up to center and pass the strap into your other hand.

2 Take the leg across your body—just a little, until you feel more stretch along the outside of the leg.

3 Keep your hip heavy on the floor and move it down, away from the shoulder on the same side so that your waist remains level. This action might feel like a side bend, but it will help you stay neutral.

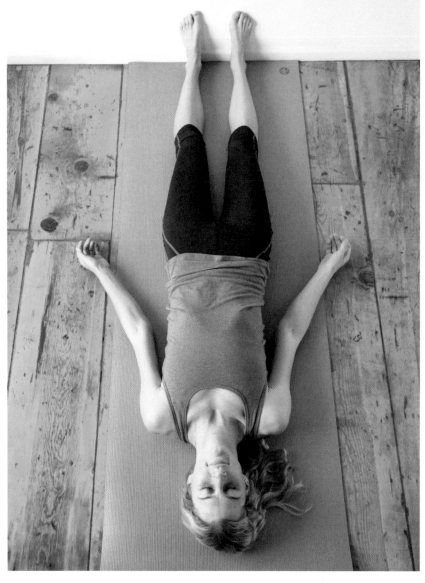

Return to Mountain at the Wall and pause to feel the difference before repeating the 3-Way Hamstrings sequence on your other side.

> " Balance is a constant and evolving adjustment toward center."
> —RICHELLE RICARD, THE YOGA ENGINEER

PAUSE AND FEEL THE DIFFERENCE

Know where stretching ends and compensation begins

Once your hamstrings reach their maximum flexibility, if you continue to pull on the strap, your spine will likely side bend to allow you to continue to move your leg toward the ceiling. This will shorten one side of your waist and make it often appear as though you've internally rotated that leg (i.e., turned your foot so that your toes point toward the center of your body).

Reality check: You're not stretching farther. While you might be getting psyched that you can get your leg farther up there, you're simply forcing another region of your body out of balance to compensate for lack of hamstring flexibility.

Rather than tug on your lifted leg, be honest about where your hamstring flexibility ends and compensation begins. Once you feel your spine and/or hips begin to shift, back off a little so that you can maintain a neutral spine and get the most benefit out of the stretch rather than push too far.

Similarly, when you do a Figure 4 at the Wall (p. 10), if you push your thigh toward the wall to deepen the stretch, your spine will side bend to keep moving the thigh forward once your hip reaches its range-of-motion limit. You're just pushing your bones around beyond their neutral alignment.

If these compensation patterns happen when you're lying down and stretching, you'd better believe they're happening when you're out running, riding, or swimming— any activity where you are lifting your legs forward and up.

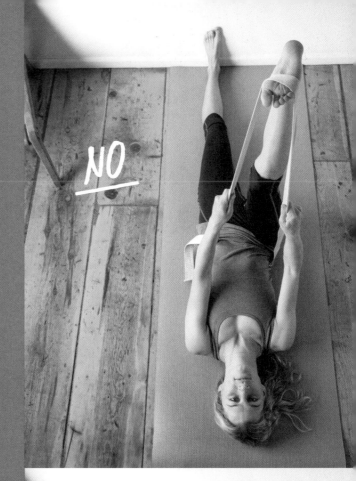

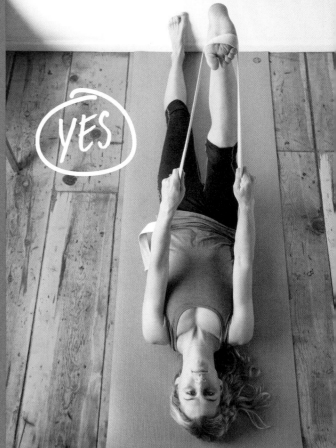

GAME PLAN

! Areas where I'm most prone
to imbalance, and why:

✔ I can mitigate my
imbalances by:

! My body compensates for
my imbalances by:

✔ My plan for five minutes
of daily yoga:

! The main things that are
impeding my balance right now:

#hitreset

✔ What are you doing to sustain balance today?

*THE LITTLE THINGS
ADD UP TO BIG THINGS
BY CREATING MORE
BALANCE IN YOUR BODY*

DO THE
**LITTLE
THINGS**

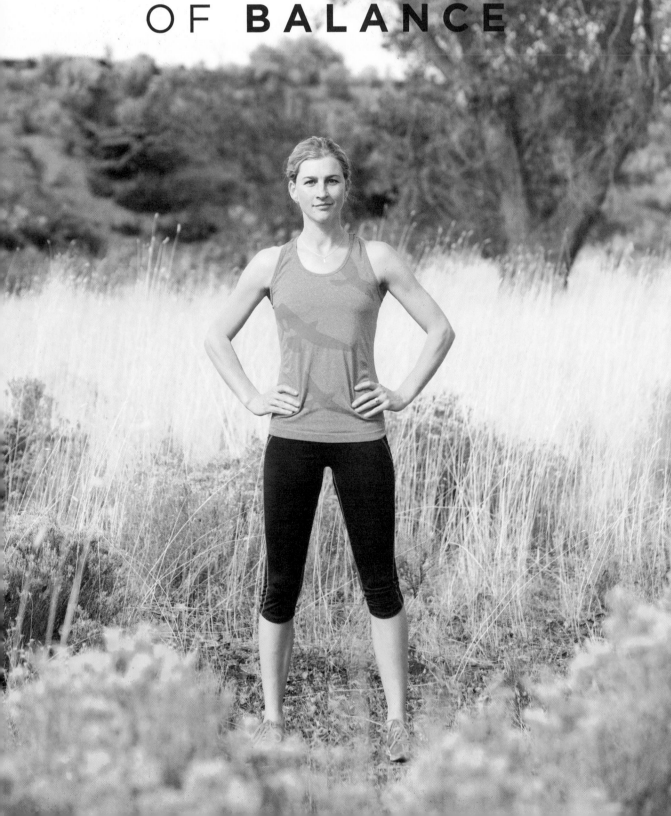

FEEL THE POWER
OF **BALANCE**

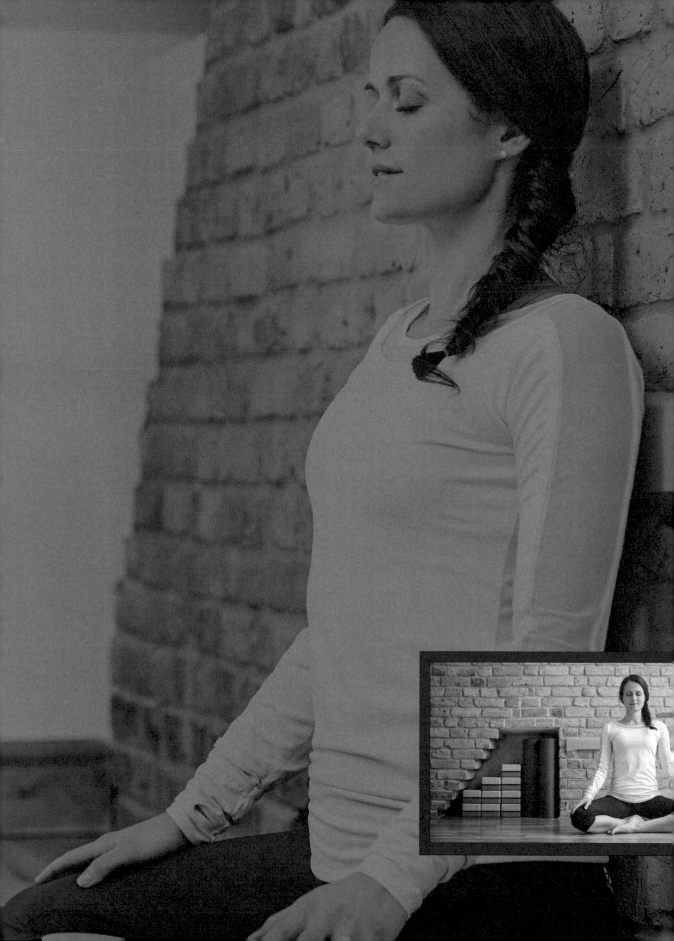

BREATHE & FOCUS

It's a good thing that you're always breathing, because your body needs oxygen to survive. But here's what you might not realize: The quality of your breath is a direct reflection of your interior state. If your breath is shallow and erratic, you're more likely to be stressed or unfocused. Breathing and mental focus are interconnected.

Your breath is powerful because it enables you to focus and relax simultaneously—these are the conditions under which you'll perform your best, no matter the task at hand. And it's accessible because no matter where you go or what you do, it's always with you.

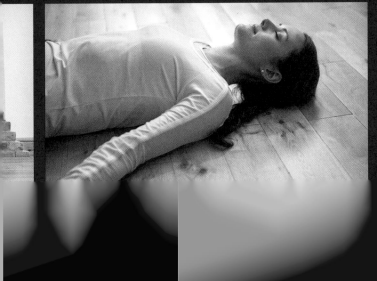

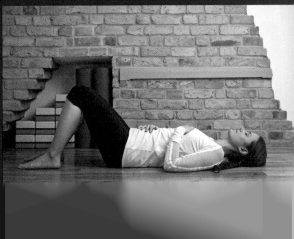

Shallow breathing = Less energy

Do you ever feel easily winded when you're working out, competing, or walking up the stairs? When you push yourself, do you find yourself holding your breath and then gasping for air? More important, are you even aware of the way in which you are breathing?

The more tired and stressed you are, the shallower your breath becomes. This causes your body to panic, resulting in more strained breathing and ultimately more fatigue. It's a vicious cycle that increases stress and decreases your endurance and performance.

✔ SOLUTION

TAKE CONTROL OF YOUR **MENTAL STATE**

Mental strength and stamina are like anything—they take practice. Conveniently, what happens on your yoga mat is a direct reflection of how you handle most things in life. As you go through different poses, use the opportunity to become more aware of your tendencies, reactions, and mental behavior. Slow down and recognize what's actually happening so that you can more readily discern how you want to respond in any given moment and how you'll manage the challenges that come at you. This is an invaluable skill at game time or in a race. It creates a baseline of steadiness that will impact everything you do.

✔ SOLUTION

FIND **BREATHING SPACE**

It's easy to lose track of your breath, especially when you're busy. You must continually remind yourself of your breath capacity. Simple breathing techniques can help you keep your cool under pressure so that your systems can function optimally, and they help you make a conscious shift from stress to relaxation. Maintaining steady breathing will also give you a boost in that last mile or in overtime.

! PROBLEM

Lack of focus inhibits performance

It doesn't matter how strong your body is if you can't focus your energy to control and coordinate your movement and stay calm and steady when challenged. If you can't silence distractions and doubt and anchor your mind on the task at hand, you risk going through the motions or choking under pressure, and you won't reach your potential.

HIT RESET
TO BREATHE & FOCUS

ROUTINES
- ✓ **Find Breathing Space** (p. 24)
- ✓ **Take Control of Your Mental State** (p. 28)

BENEFITS

> Become aware of your breathing so you can use it to full advantage

> Sharpen mental focus

PRACTICE	Pre-workout/crosstraining Post-workout/recovery
PROPS	Bolster, pillow, or folded blanket to sit on
RED FLAGS	Spinal compensation via rounding forward General discomfort that inhibits your ability to focus

YOUR BREATH IS YOUR MOST POWERFUL AND ACCESSIBLE TOOL

FAQ How do I stop stressing about time?

If your schedule is tight or going watchless makes you sweat, set a timer for however much time you want to spend on your breathing and focusing practices so you don't have to wonder what time it is. Approach whatever amount of time you decide to spend here as a break—a Reset.

TECHNIQUE

For starters:
Get comfortable

It's really important to find a comfortable setup for your breathing and focusing practices. This helps to eliminate distraction and makes it easier to be present rather than aching everywhere and dying for it to be over. There are a few great ways to accomplish this:

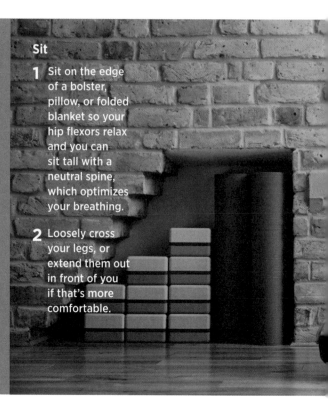

Sit

1 Sit on the edge of a bolster, pillow, or folded blanket so your hip flexors relax and you can sit tall with a neutral spine, which optimizes your breathing.

2 Loosely cross your legs, or extend them out in front of you if that's more comfortable.

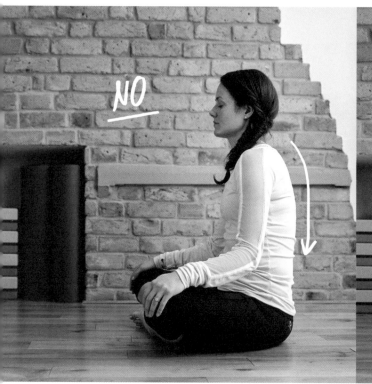

NO

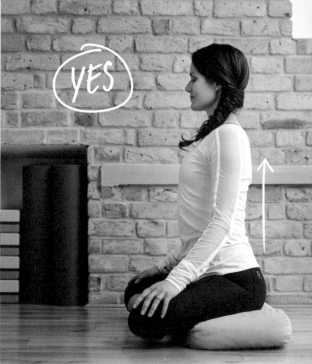

YES

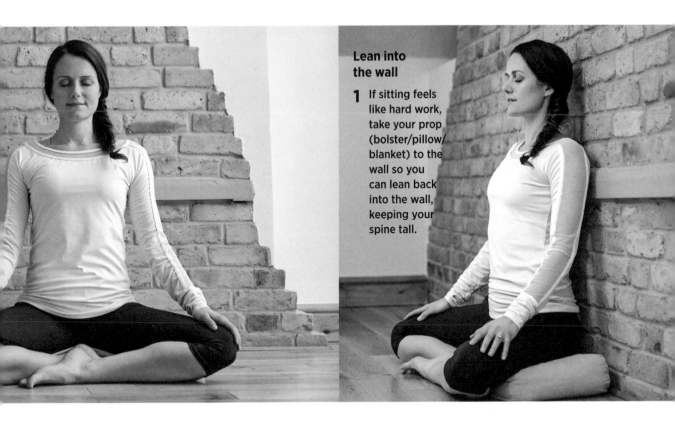

Lean into the wall

1 If sitting feels like hard work, take your prop (bolster/pillow/blanket) to the wall so you can lean back into the wall, keeping your spine tall.

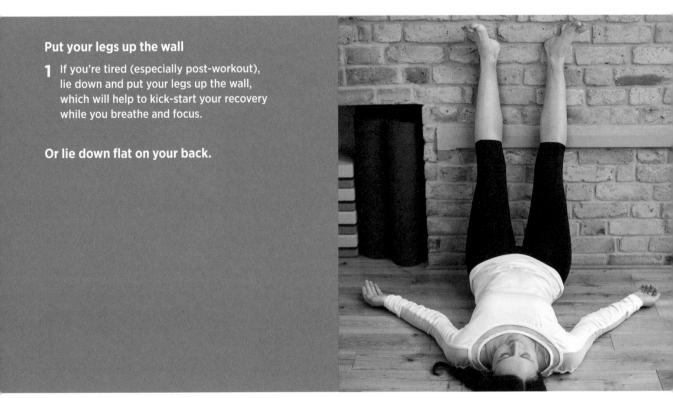

Put your legs up the wall

1 If you're tired (especially post-workout), lie down and put your legs up the wall, which will help to kick-start your recovery while you breathe and focus.

Or lie down flat on your back.

✔ FIND **BREATHING SPACE**

MATCHING BREATH

1 Take a deep breath in … a slow breath out.

2 Inhale as you count 1–2–3–4 …

3 Exhale as you count 1–2–3–4.

4 Breathe in for 4 …

5 And out for 4.

6 Keep slowing it down, and see if you can lengthen your count to 5 or 6, or more.

7 Continue for 2–5 minutes.

THE QUALITY OF YOUR BREATH WILL TELL YOU EXACTLY WHAT YOU NEED TO KNOW ABOUT YOUR INTERIOR STATE

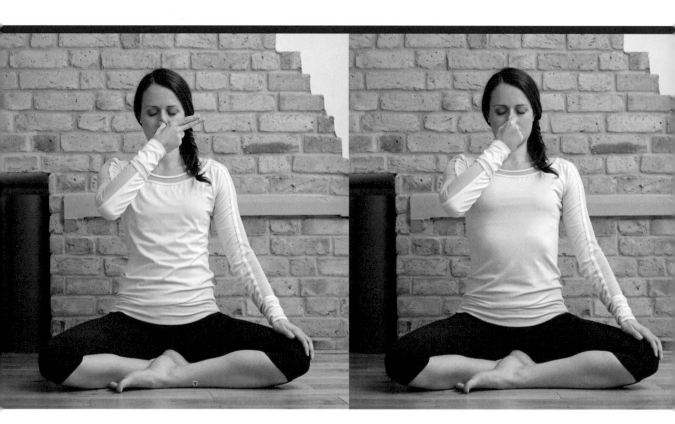

WARRIOR BREATH

1 Take a deep breath in … a slow breath out.

2 Inhale through your nose … then exhale out your mouth as if you're trying to fog up a window with your breath.

3 On your next breath, do the same thing except with your mouth closed—creating an audible wavelike sound as you breathe in and out through your nose.

4 Continue for 2–5 minutes.

STAY WITH IT!

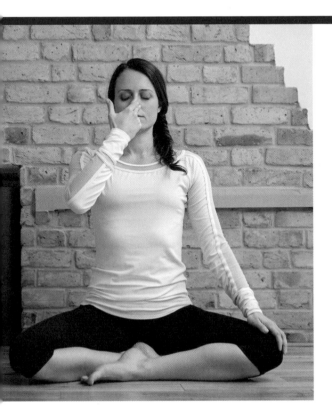

BALANCING BREATH

1 Hold one hand in front of your face—curl your pinky and ring fingers into your palm, leaving your middle and pointer fingers and thumb out.

2 Take a deep breath in … a slow breath out.

3 Cover one nostril with your thumb and slowly inhale through your other nostril …

4 Close your other nostril with your free fingers and pause …

5 Remove your thumb and slowly exhale through that side.

6 Keeping your finger-side nostril closed, inhale through the thumb-side nostril …

7 Close the thumb-side nostril and pause …

8 Open your finger-side nostril and exhale to complete one round.

9 Continue slowly for 5 rounds.

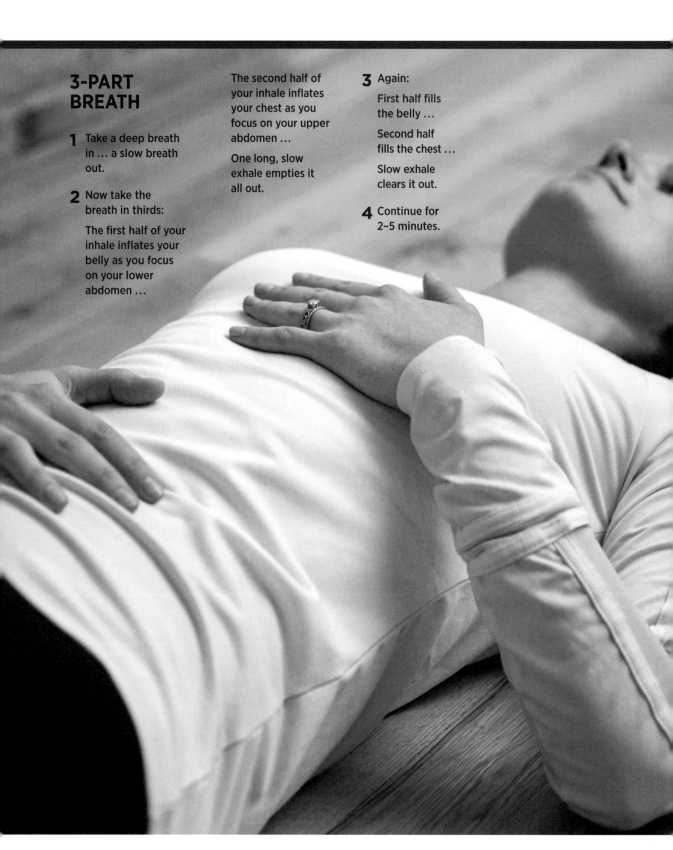

3-PART BREATH

1 Take a deep breath in ... a slow breath out.

2 Now take the breath in thirds:

The first half of your inhale inflates your belly as you focus on your lower abdomen ...

The second half of your inhale inflates your chest as you focus on your upper abdomen ...

One long, slow exhale empties it all out.

3 Again:

First half fills the belly ...

Second half fills the chest ...

Slow exhale clears it out.

4 Continue for 2–5 minutes.

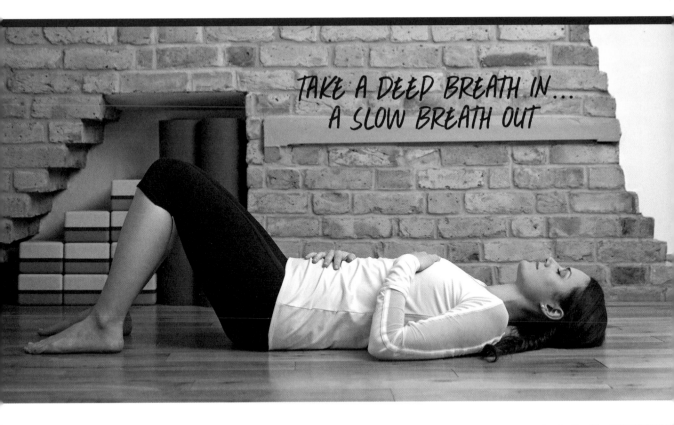

TAKE A DEEP BREATH IN...
A SLOW BREATH OUT

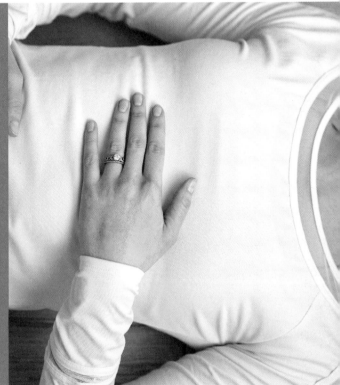

TECHNIQUE
Gather feedback

If feeling where your breath is moving seems elusive, put your hands on your torso, which will give you more feedback. Place one hand just below your navel, the other on your chest. Or, to help direct your breath somewhere else, put a hand on that spot. Feel your breath move beneath your hands.

BE HERE NOW

In sports and in life, mantras—positive affirmations—are helpful because they anchor you in the present and cut through any chaos, doubt, or negativity in your head. They can help you manage any challenge more easefully.

1 Take a deep breath in … a slow breath out.

2 Inhaling, say in your head, "I am … "

3 Exhaling, say, "here now."

4 Inhale: "I am … "

5 Exhale: "here now."

6 Continue for 2–5 minutes, and feel free to replace this mantra with any positive phrase that resonates with you!

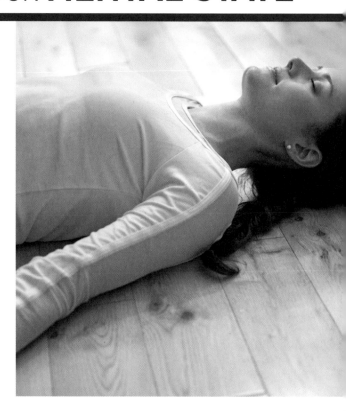

FEEL THE FEELING OF ACHIEVING YOUR GOAL

Not just thinking but truly feeling your goals as already achieved creates a powerful bridge between where you are now and where you want to be.

1 Take a deep breath in … a slow breath out. Continue to deepen your breathing.

2 Once your breath feels steady, begin to focus on your goal—if a few things come to mind, try to focus on one specific thing.

3 Once you have that clear goal in your mind, shift your focus away from the goal itself, considering instead how achieving that goal would make you feel. How would you feel different? Would you be more confident? Feel more fulfilled?

4 Focus not on the goal itself but on the resulting feelings, and notice the sensations in your body.

5 Sit with that until the feeling is clear and realistic.

6 Now refocus on your goal from the perspective of someone who has already accomplished it.

7 Then open your eyes and carry that confidence—that belief in your ability to manifest that goal—with you, as if you have already accomplished it.

If the feeling you seek is elusive, it's no big deal. The more you practice and the more you begin to believe in your ability to achieve your goal, the more readily you'll be able to access that feeling. Be patient with yourself—stay with it!

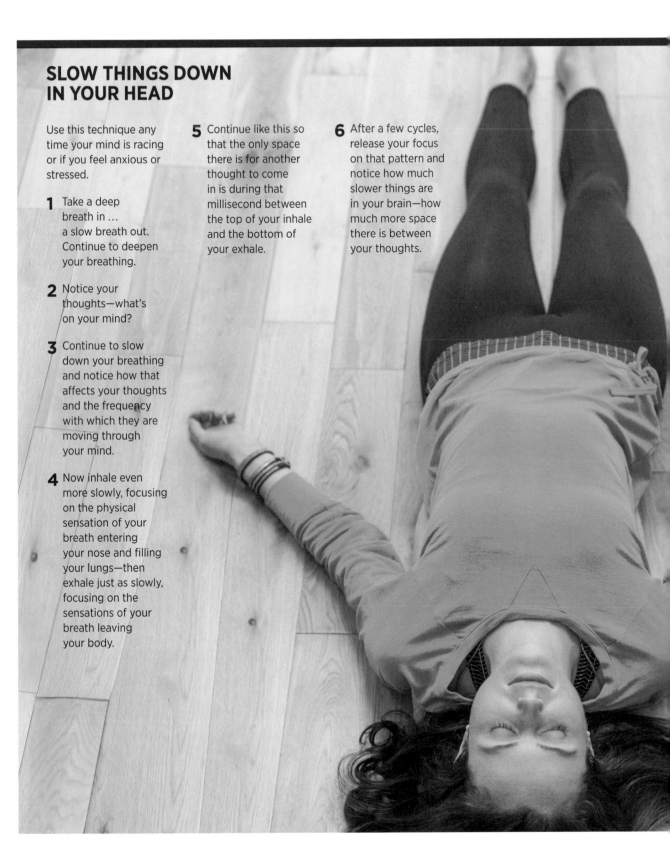

SLOW THINGS DOWN IN YOUR HEAD

Use this technique any time your mind is racing or if you feel anxious or stressed.

1 Take a deep breath in … a slow breath out. Continue to deepen your breathing.

2 Notice your thoughts—what's on your mind?

3 Continue to slow down your breathing and notice how that affects your thoughts and the frequency with which they are moving through your mind.

4 Now inhale even more slowly, focusing on the physical sensation of your breath entering your nose and filling your lungs—then exhale just as slowly, focusing on the sensations of your breath leaving your body.

5 Continue like this so that the only space there is for another thought to come in is during that millisecond between the top of your inhale and the bottom of your exhale.

6 After a few cycles, release your focus on that pattern and notice how much slower things are in your brain—how much more space there is between your thoughts.

GAME
PLAN

! My breath becomes erratic when:

✔ When things get crazy, I'll breathe like this to stay calm:

! It's hard for me to focus when:

✔ I will sharpen my mental focus by:

#hitreset

✔ What are you doing to breathe and focus better today?

PAY ATTENTION

DO THE
**LITTLE
THINGS**

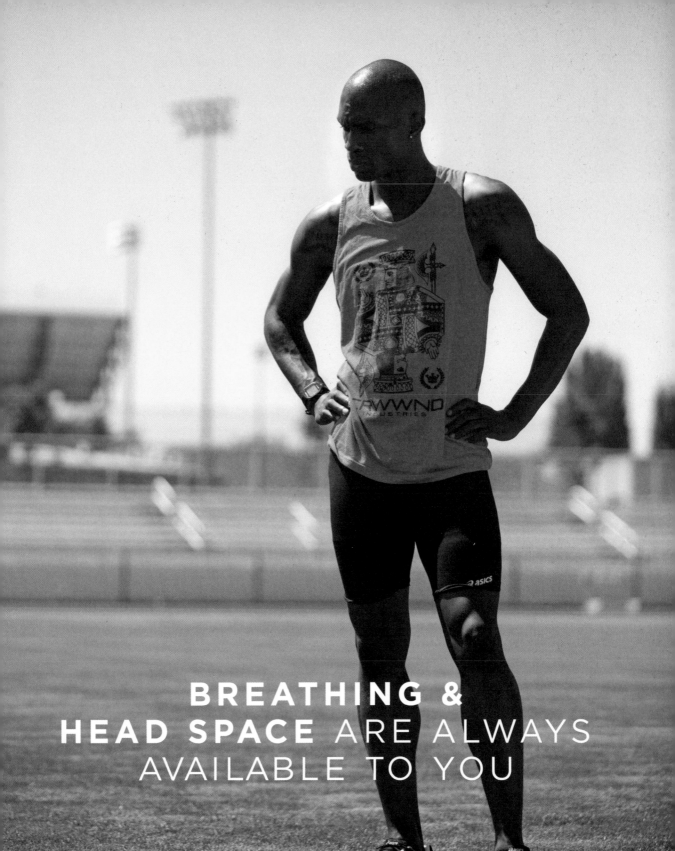

**BREATHING &
HEAD SPACE** ARE ALWAYS
AVAILABLE TO YOU

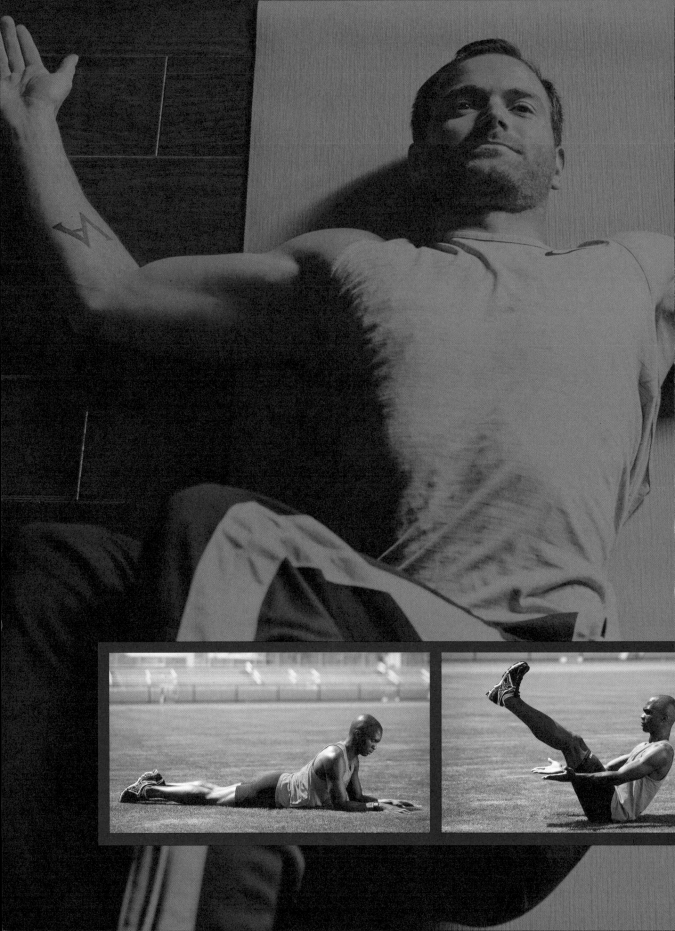

STRENGTHEN
YOUR CORE

Your core is the engine for your extremities. It is, fundamentally, your powerhouse.

While most people aspire to a lean, toned midsection, a buff bod doesn't necessarily equate to a strong core. A six-pack might look nice, but those surface-level abs are pretty useless when it comes to maintaining good posture, avoiding back pain, or helping you avoid falling while you fly down the mountain on your bike or skis.

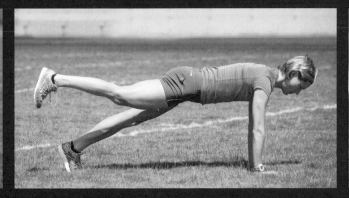
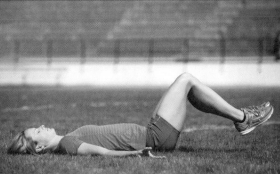

Sleepy center limits your power

The most important layer of your abdominal muscles—your transverse—lives deep in your abdomen. It wraps around your midsection kind of like a corset, stabilizes your spine, and adds power to all your movements.

The problem is that athletes tend to go through the motions of doing core work without awareness that the transverse is even in there. And if you're not aware of a muscle or how to activate it, you can't effectively strengthen it or use it to full advantage.

More than anything, that deep layer of muscle is sleepy from sitting all day long. Think about it: Aside from your fave sports and fitness activities, what do you do a lot of? You sit. All the time—in your car, at your desk, at breakfast/lunch/dinner, on your couch … you get the point. And what do sitting and most workouts have in common? They both result in stiffness across the chest (hips too, but let's focus on upper body for now). It doesn't help that a lot of core work is like a compensation free-for-all—it isn't particularly effective for training the transverse, nor is it particularly functional. Exercises like crunches make it easy to cheat by using momentum and arm strength to drive movement. In addition, when you lie on your back and round your upper torso forward off the floor to do a crunch, you're simply reinforcing the bad posture you've spent all day cultivating. Over time, you'll continue to strain your neck, overstretch your upper back, and slouch forward even more. The fact is you don't need help rounding forward because chances are you're already there.

✔ SOLUTION

TURN ON YOUR
TRANSVERSE

A strong transverse that can stabilize your spine in neutral—especially when you're tired—will optimize your power and help you avoid injuries. What's your most common movement pattern? Walking, running, or anything forward-oriented. So working your core while mimicking that movement will help you wrap your mind around how to engage those muscles while you're actually out walking and running around, riding your bike, and even sitting at your desk.

! PROBLEM

Weak obliques fail to stabilize & twist

You have two sets of obliques, on both the right and left side of your trunk, which are known as the internal and external obliques. Not quite as deep as the transverse, they're responsible for twisting your spine, and when you engage both the right and left simultaneously, they provide stability—they make it feel like your front ribs are moving toward each other, as if you're going to knit the front of your rib cage closed.

The problem is that some people's bodies naturally love extension—back bending— which isn't surprising given that the mid-spine is the most mobile part of your back. Extension lovers are essentially the opposite of the forward floppers discussed above. It's like this: If you lean your torso back, you'll feel your front ribs on your right and left move farther away from each other, as if your rib cage is expanding. Imagine you're reaching overhead to serve a tennis ball or volleyball. If you don't counter the action of reaching up by engaging your core to keep your spine stable, you're putting yourself at risk for compensation and injury.

Additionally, if you're not using your obliques to drive your rotation, you're most definitely relying on momentum, arm strength, or a combination of both. The bicycle crunch is a classic example of this, where you twist to take your elbow toward the opposite knee while crunching.

✔ SOLUTION

[STABILIZE & TWIST]

It's easy to use arm strength and momentum to twist your upper body. It takes way more focus to use your obliques to twist, but it's worth the effort because you'll gain power and avoid back pain and injuries. Strengthen the muscles that keep your mid-spine stable—slow down and make them do the work to rotate your trunk.

STOP FLAILING AND START WORKING!

Weak back can't hold you upright

Let's talk about your most fundamental back core muscle for a second: quadratus lumborum, also known as QL. Along with the smaller muscles that live along your spine, this guy plays a key role in helping you sit up straight rather than rounding your low back.

The problem again is sitting, the effects of which are amplified when we go to work out. After slouching over your desk all day and then slouching over the elliptical machine, guess what? Your back is overstretched and weak. Most people don't realize this. You might feel sore around your low back, but it's more likely that area is pissed off because your core has been asleep all day and your back is tired from being overstretched. It's the opposite of what you might think is going on back there. But let's be real: When was the last time you complained about your weak core, which is really to blame for your aching back?

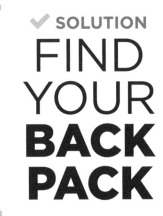

✔ SOLUTION

FIND YOUR **BACK PACK**

All this talk about six-packs … what about your back pack? Your back pack isn't just the area of your trunk directly opposite to your six-pack. Your key back core muscles—your back pack—span pretty much the entire length of your trunk. These guys have to be strong to support optimal posture, stabilize your spine, and prevent back pain. Work 'em!

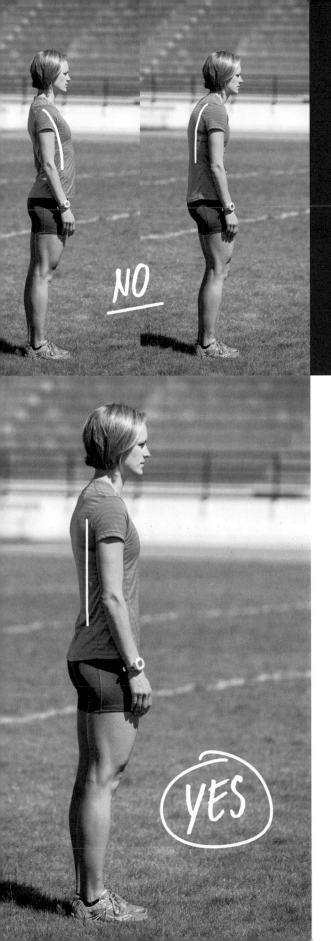

WHERE'S YOUR CORE WEAKNESS?

Stand in profile in front of a mirror and observe your posture. (You can also do this test sitting on the floor, which isolates the issue even more.)

✔ CORRECT

> **If your weight shifts forward and your rib cage wants to pop open:** This is a good sign that your obliques are weak and you will benefit from the Stabilize & Twist routine (p. 46).

> **If your back rounds, making it tough to maintain an upright posture:** This signals that you lack back strength, which you can remedy with the Find Your Back Pack routine (p. 50).

> **For everyone:** It's safe to assume that your transverse could use some work, so be sure to hit up the Turn On Your Transverse routine (p. 40).

HIT RESET TO STRENGTHEN YOUR CORE

ROUTINES

✔ **Turn On Your Transverse** (p. 40)

✔ **Stabilize & Twist** (p. 46)

✔ **Find Your Back Pack** (p. 50)

BENEFITS

> Become aware of, activate, and strengthen your core muscles so you can use them to full advantage

> Improve posture

> Prevent low back pain and compensation injuries

> Add power to all movement

PRACTICE	Pre-workout/crosstraining
HOW LONG	Hold for 3–5 breaths or 10+ reps/multiple sets for movement
PROPS	Block and bolster, pillow, or folded blanket
RED FLAGS	Spinal compensation via back bending or side bending Neck and shoulder strain

TECHNIQUE
Work from neutral

1 Lie on your back with your knees bent and your feet on the floor.

2 Do a few cat/cows into the floor—arch and round your low back while keeping your butt on the floor to feel the range of movement available to you.

3 Eventually stop in the middle, the even point between the two extremes of arching and rounding your spine—keep your spine there.

4 Now put your hands onto your waist and feel an equal amount of space between your ribs and hips on both your right and left sides—make sure your spine isn't side bending. Lift up your head and look if you need more feedback about where your body is in space.

>> The body easily forgets where center is, so use these simple tools (cat/cow to find the right position for your low back, and hands on your torso to feel for even space between your ribs and hips on both sides) whenever you need a reminder.

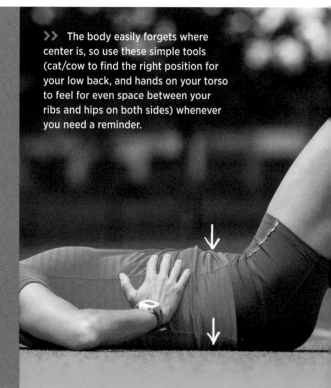

FAQ **How do I engage my core?**

When it comes to engaging your core, you should be thinking about your transverse. Not sure if it's awake? Here's a tool to clarify:

> Bring your hands onto your waist between your ribs and hips.

> Cough!

> Feel that contraction under your hands when you cough? Those are your deep abdominal muscles—your transverse and obliques, too.

> Now see if you can create that same contraction without coughing and hold it without holding your breath.

> You should feel engagement around your low belly as well as your rib cage—if that's elusive, focus on bringing your front ribs closer together, as if you're trying to knit them together.

> When all this is engaged, it should feel a bit like you've put on a tight vest.

> As you keep that engagement through your center, you should feel as if you're able to lengthen your spine.

> Remember, when in doubt about whether your core is firing, cough!

EQUAL SPACE BETWEEN
YOUR RIBS AND HIPS = STABLE CORE

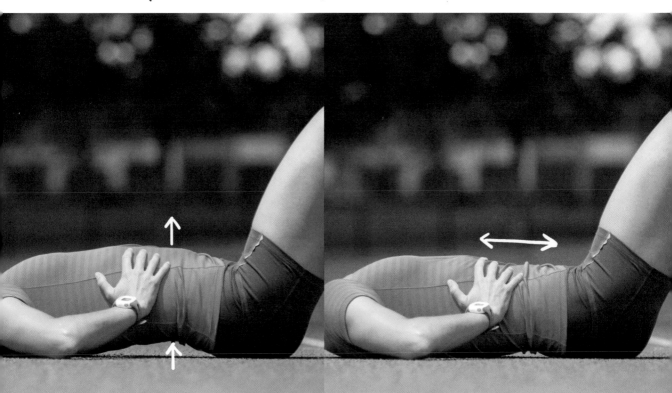

✔ TURN ON YOUR **TRANSVERSE**

TABLE TOP

1 Lie on your back with your knees bent, feet hip width apart on the floor, and lengthen your arms along your sides, palms facing up.

2 Bring your spine to neutral and without letting your low back move, lift your legs to bring your knees over your hips at a 90-degree angle.

3 Engage your core to stabilize your spine in neutral as you hold your legs there, as if you're pulling your belly down toward your spine.

Relax your hip flexors—take the work out of your legs and put it into your core.

LIFT & LOWER

1 Set up Table Top and keep your knees bent at 90 degrees throughout the movement.

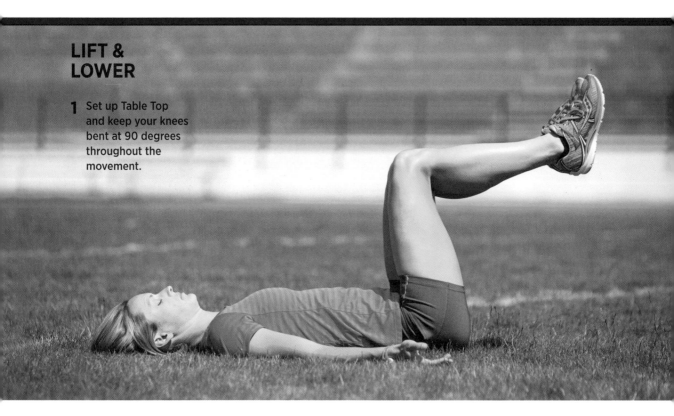

TECHNIQUE
Make a unileg

Why add a block? It's like this: Your pelvis and your legs are three pieces, and if you go blockless, you've got three pieces to coordinate. When you have a block or something to squeeze between your thighs, then you only have two parts to coordinate—your unileg and your pelvis—which is way easier to stabilize and a great place to start. If you feel your low back straining, or you find it difficult to keep your lifted legs side by side, gently squeeze a block between your upper inner thighs for the Table Top and Lift & Lower poses to create more stability.

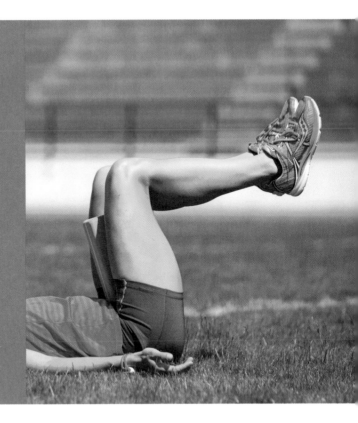

2 Lower the legs a few inches forward toward the floor, keeping your core engaged and your spine neutral—if you feel your low back arch, the movement is too big.

3 Bring your knees back up over your hips.

4 Continue, using your core to stabilize your spine while you move your legs.

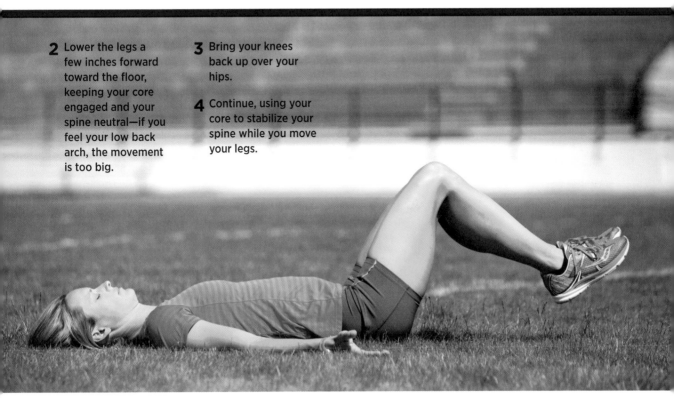

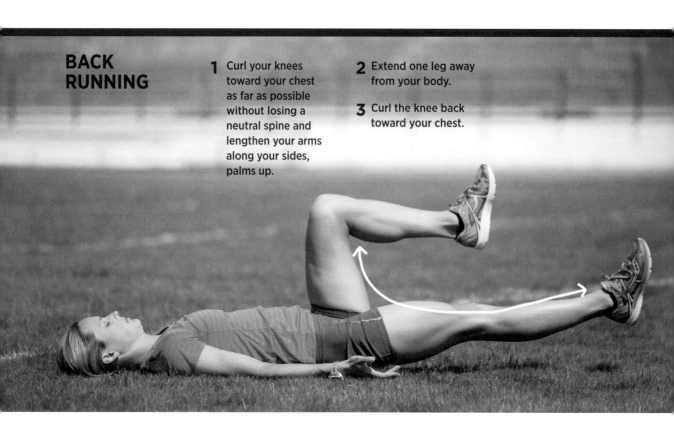

BACK RUNNING

1 Curl your knees toward your chest as far as possible without losing a neutral spine and lengthen your arms along your sides, palms up.

2 Extend one leg away from your body.

3 Curl the knee back toward your chest.

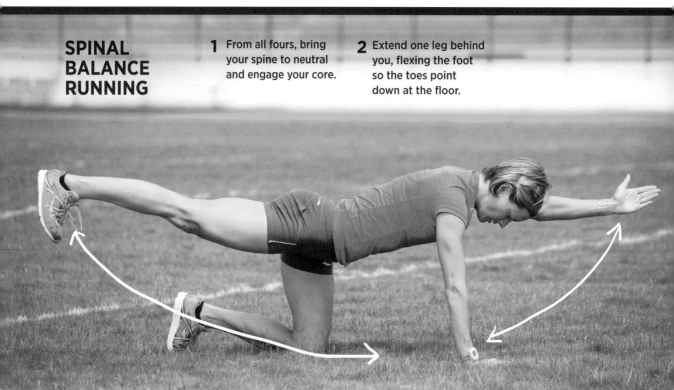

SPINAL BALANCE RUNNING

1 From all fours, bring your spine to neutral and engage your core.

2 Extend one leg behind you, flexing the foot so the toes point down at the floor.

4 Extend your other leg away from your body.

5 Curl the knee toward your chest.

6 Continue, using your core to stabilize your spine while you move your legs.

>> When you feel strong and stable in this movement, you can make it more fluid, as if you're walking, running, or cycling.

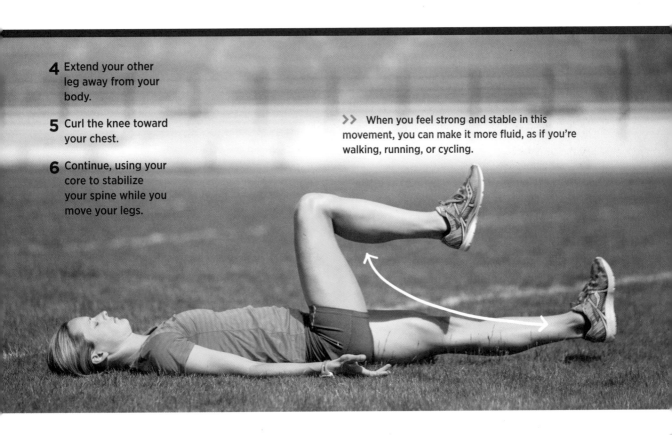

3 Reach your opposite arm forward alongside your ear, thumb pointing up.

4 Without moving your spine, bring your lifted knee and elbow toward each other.

5 Reextend your leg and arm.

6 Continue, keeping your spine stable.

Repeat on your other side.

>> Resist the urge to bring your elbow and knee together, as that will round your spine out of neutral.

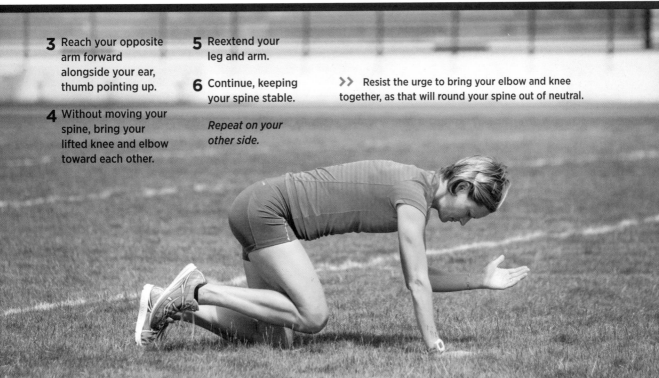

PLANK

1 Come to all fours with your hands flat to the floor and step your legs back into a push-up position, toes tucked under.

2 Engage your core to stabilize your spine in neutral by lifting from your low belly and front ribs.

3 Push back through your toes and forward through your hands, helping to integrate your extremities.

Don't slip into banana back.

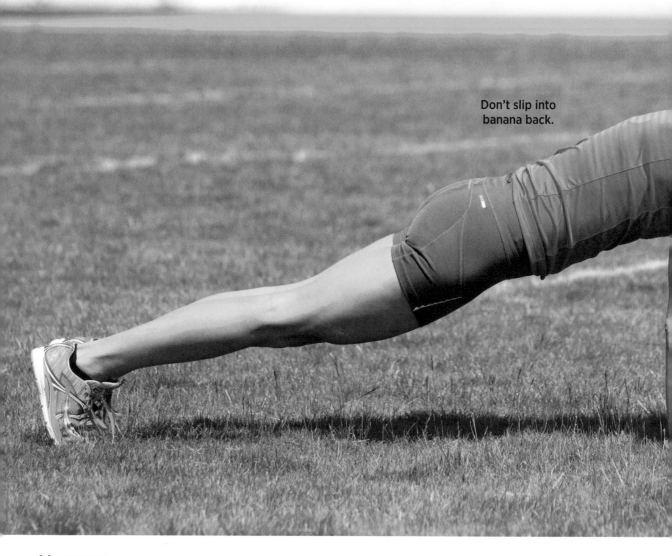

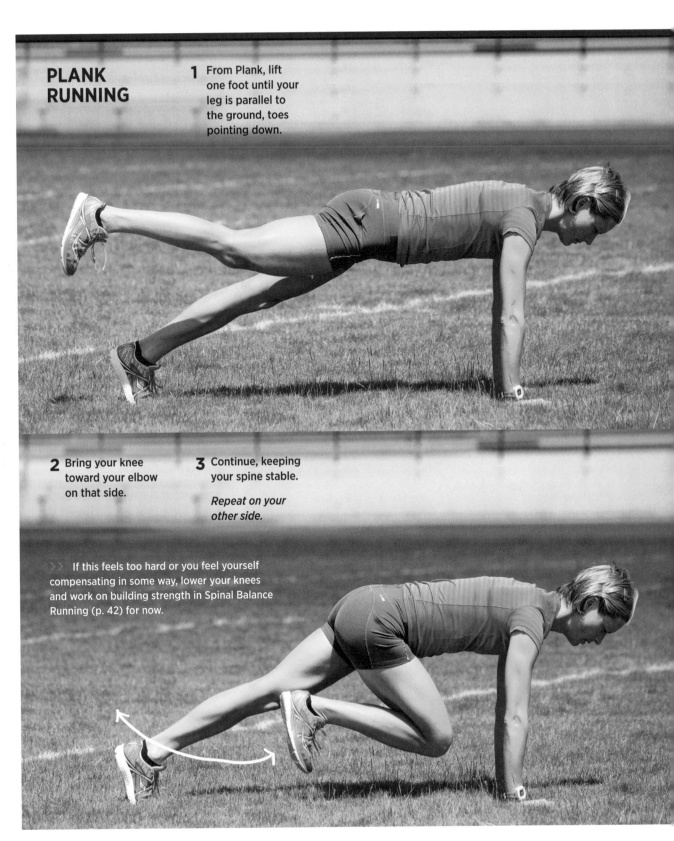

PLANK RUNNING

1 From Plank, lift one foot until your leg is parallel to the ground, toes pointing down.

2 Bring your knee toward your elbow on that side.

3 Continue, keeping your spine stable.

Repeat on your other side.

>> If this feels too hard or you feel yourself compensating in some way, lower your knees and work on building strength in Spinal Balance Running (p. 42) for now.

STABILIZE & TWIST

SEATED TWISTING

1 Sit cross-legged, on your shins, or with your legs extended out in front of you—if it's tough to sit up straight, sit on a bolster/pillow/folded blanket.

2 Join your palms in front of your chest.

3 Engage your core to lengthen your spine.

4 Twist as far as you can to one side, using only your core (rather than momentum or arm strength) and keeping everything below your rib cage still so that only your rib cage is rotating on the axis of your spine.

5 Return to center and twist to the other side.

6 Continue …

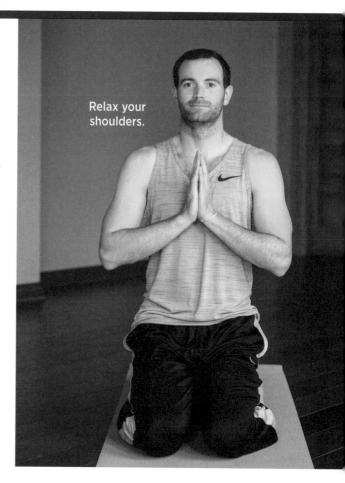

Relax your shoulders.

BONUS For the crunch junkies

Sorry, crunch junkies, but the time has come to ditch the limb-flailing, torso-jerking, neck-straining mainstay of traditional ab work.

Here's why: All the sitting you do over computers, steering wheels, and plates of food encourages your shoulders to round forward, which pretty much makes your body default into hunch mode. Since you don't need help flopping forward, crunch your body from extension (back bend) to neutral—in doing so you'll build more practical core strength and keep your body more balanced.

If you must crunch, crunch like this:

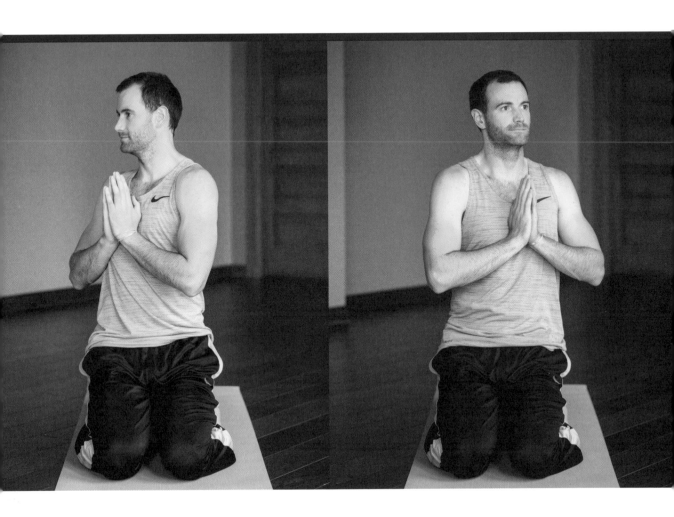

CRUNCH OVER BOLSTER

1 Sit down and place a bolster or a few stacked pillows or folded blankets at the bottom of your shoulder blades, horizontally.

2 Bend your knees, put your feet on the floor, and lie back over your props—you should be in a pretty big back bend with your mid-spine on the props (adjust if needed).

3 Support the back of your head/base of your skull with inter-laced fingers, keeping your elbows wide.

4 Engage your core and lift your spine up to neutral.

5 Lower to the start.

6 Continue …

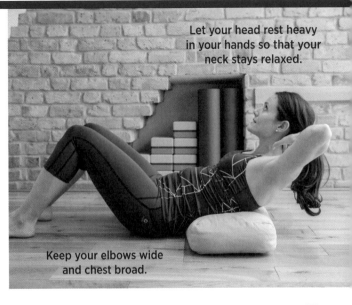

Let your head rest heavy in your hands so that your neck stays relaxed.

Keep your elbows wide and chest broad.

SIDE TO SIDE

1 Set up Table Top (p. 40) and keep your knees bent throughout the movement.

2 Lower the legs a few inches toward one side.

3 Bring your knees back up over your hips.

4 Lower the legs a few inches toward the other side.

5 Bring your knees back up over your hips.

6 Continue, using your core to control the movement of your legs.

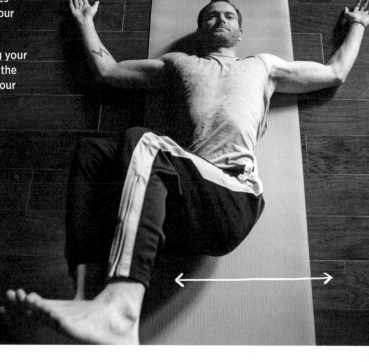

ROLL BACK ROTATION

1 Sit with your legs straight in front of you on the floor and reach your arms out in front of you. Sit on a folded blanket if it's hard to sit up tall.

2 Keeping your spine long, lean back a little.

3 Lengthen your spine.

4 Rotate your rib cage and arms to one side, without moving your legs.

5 Return to center.

6 Rotate your rib cage and arms to the other side, without moving your legs.

7 Return to center.

8 Lean back farther and repeat two more rounds before releasing all the way down to the floor.

>> To help keep your hips still while you work on rotating your upper body, reach for that block again.

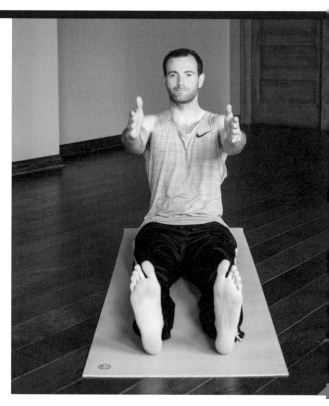

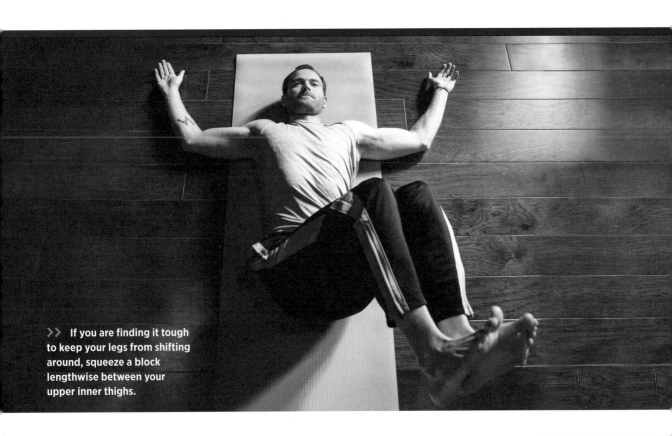

>> If you are finding it tough to keep your legs from shifting around, squeeze a block lengthwise between your upper inner thighs.

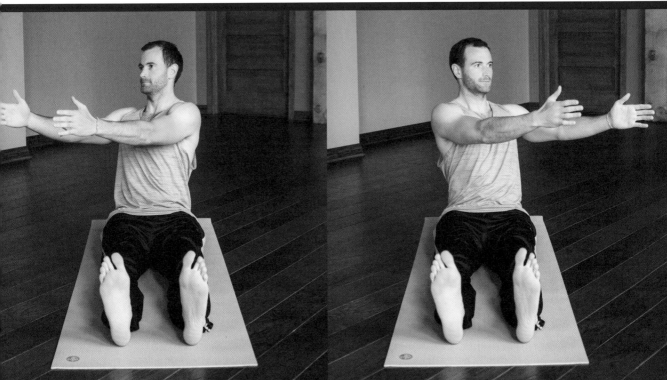

✔ FIND YOUR **BACK PACK**

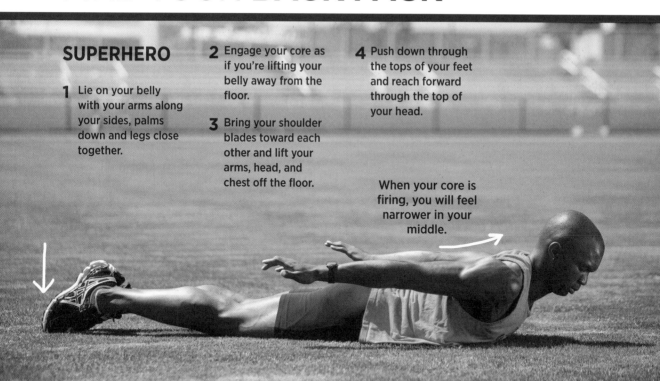

SUPERHERO

1 Lie on your belly with your arms along your sides, palms down and legs close together.

2 Engage your core as if you're lifting your belly away from the floor.

3 Bring your shoulder blades toward each other and lift your arms, head, and chest off the floor.

4 Push down through the tops of your feet and reach forward through the top of your head.

When your core is firing, you will feel narrower in your middle.

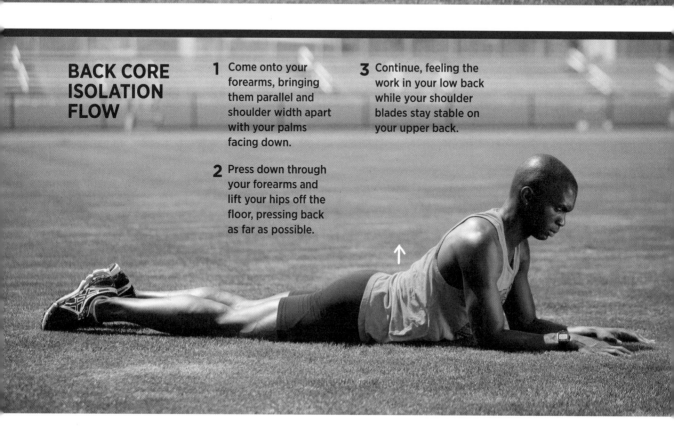

BACK CORE ISOLATION FLOW

1 Come onto your forearms, bringing them parallel and shoulder width apart with your palms facing down.

2 Press down through your forearms and lift your hips off the floor, pressing back as far as possible.

3 Continue, feeling the work in your low back while your shoulder blades stay stable on your upper back.

BACK CORE ISOLATION

1 Come onto your forearms, bringing them parallel and shoulder width apart with your palms facing down.

2 Squeeze your shoulder blades together.

3 Engage your core and focus on bringing your ribs together, as if you're trying to knit your front ribs together while simultaneously lengthening your chest forward.

4 Hold that engagement and lift your belly another inch above the floor, and hold.

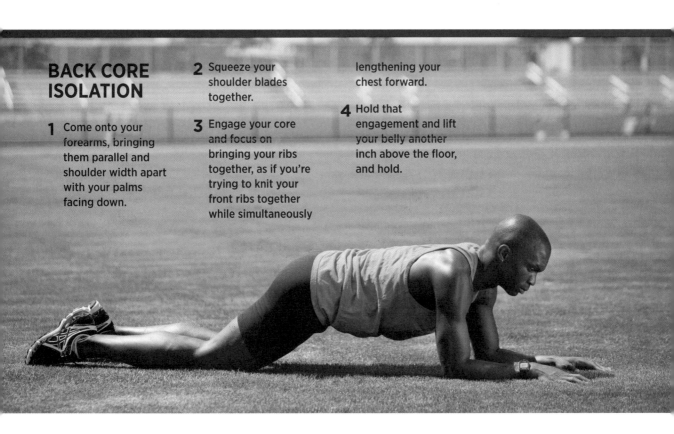

▶▶ Once you feel super strong and stable in Back Core Isolation, you're ready for Boat. If you're able to avoid rounding your low back, you are up to the challenge of Boat.

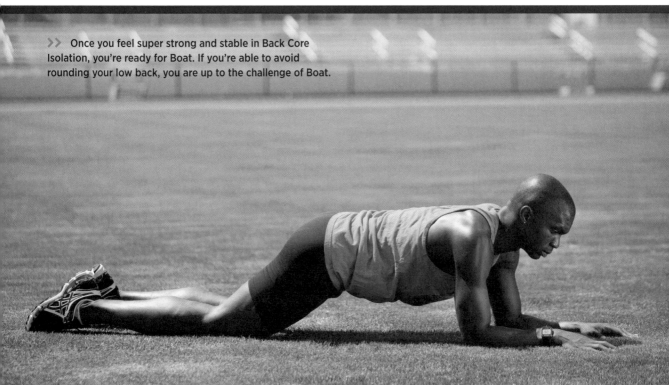

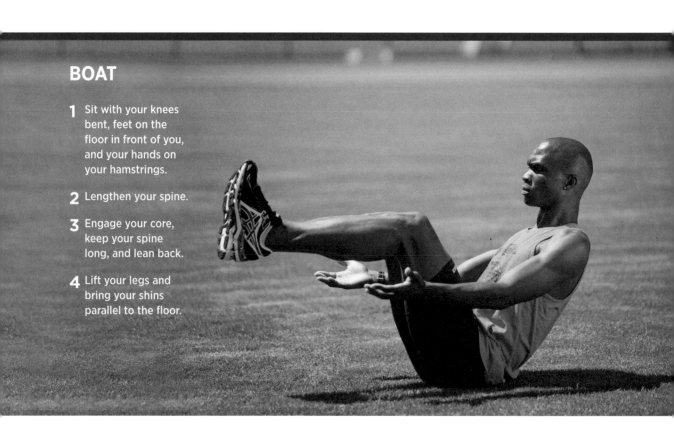

BOAT

1 Sit with your knees bent, feet on the floor in front of you, and your hands on your hamstrings.

2 Lengthen your spine.

3 Engage your core, keep your spine long, and lean back.

4 Lift your legs and bring your shins parallel to the floor.

SPINAL BALANCE

1 From all fours, bring your spine to neutral and engage your core.

2 Extend one leg behind you, flexing the foot so the toes point down at the floor.

3 Reach your opposite arm forward alongside your ear, thumb pointing up.

4 Reach longer back through the lifted heel and forward through the lifted hand.

Repeat on your other side.

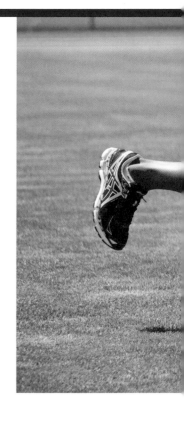

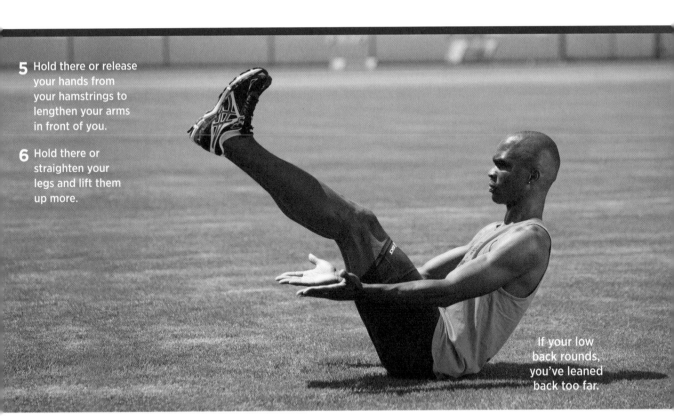

5 Hold there or release your hands from your hamstrings to lengthen your arms in front of you.

6 Hold there or straighten your legs and lift them up more.

If your low back rounds, you've leaned back too far.

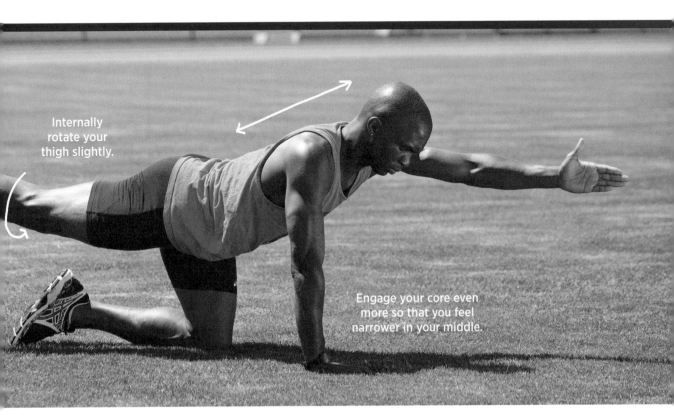

Internally rotate your thigh slightly.

Engage your core even more so that you feel narrower in your middle.

GAME
PLAN

! My spine/posture compensates for my core imbalance by:

! This affects my sports movement/ performance by:

✔ The core pose that will help me the most is: ← *DO AS MUCH AS POSSIBLE!*

#hitreset

✔ What are you doing to strengthen your core today?

BUILD YOUR CORE STRENGTH FROM THE INSIDE OUT

DO THE
**LITTLE
THINGS**

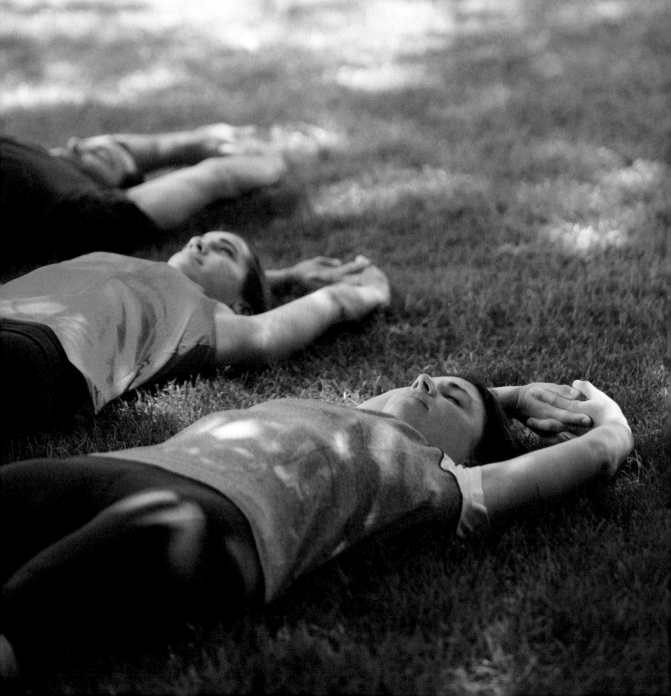

AFTER YOU'VE DONE
ALL THAT, THIS WILL
FEEL AMAZING

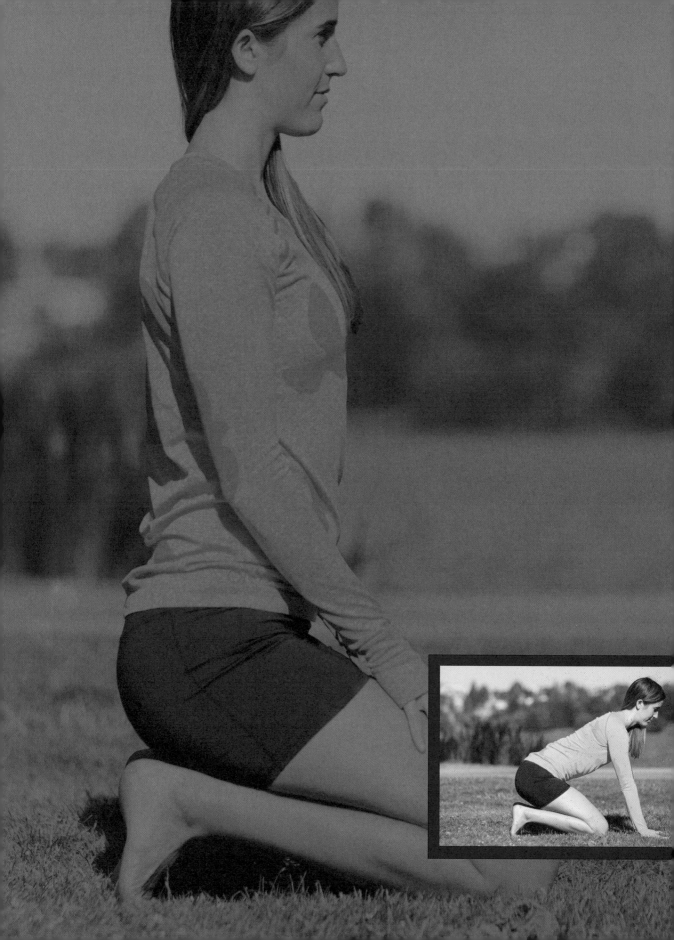

BALANCE *YOUR* FOUNDATION

It all starts in your feet. They're your foundation and they play a significant role in how your other joints align, yet those poor guys get very little attention. Unfortunately, most of us aren't very aware of our feet and toes, which isn't surprising given that we wear super-cushioned sneakers most of the time.

Also worth noting is the intimate relationship between your feet and the entire structure of your lower legs, because it's not uncommon for foot problems to originate in your lower legs, and vice versa.

While your instinct post-workout might be to direct all your attention to more obvious areas of stiffness such as hips and hamstrings, your foundation is equally important, and neglecting it will put you at risk.

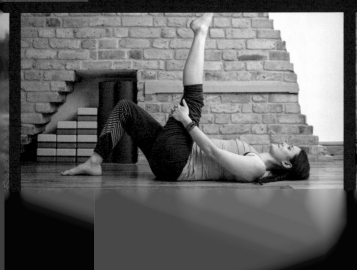
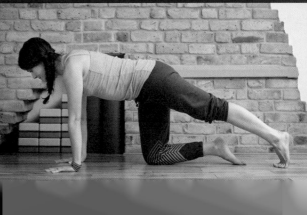

Sleepy feet are unstable

You can't really blame your feet for sleeping since you wear shoes all the time. While they're hanging out in all that cushion, your toes get stuck together. Consider this: Your big toe is meant to provide about 80–85 percent of the primary support to your foot. How's that toe supposed to do its job if you don't have any control over it? Exactly. The muscles that stabilize your arches also become lazy, and you lose finite control of the small intrinsic muscles—less prominent muscles that provide stability, kind of like little helpers— that are critical for optimal function. This decreases your ability to absorb shock while walking or running, further increasing your injury risk.

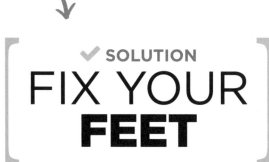

✔ SOLUTION

FIX YOUR FEET

It's true that there are different types of feet with different injury patterns, so there's no perfect solution for everyone. But you'll have no idea what's going on down there unless you kick your kicks off and start paying attention. In general, your arches should be active and your toes should be like monkey toes— you should have some control over them (be able to intentionally spread them out and wiggle them around). Building strength, increasing fluidity, and gaining control of your toes and feet will help you to use them optimally and avoid injuries.

❝ *Shoes don't stabilize the arch. Muscles do—train 'em!"*

—JAY DICHARRY, PHYSICAL THERAPIST AND RESEARCHER

Stiff calves lack fluidity

Your calves are compartmentalized structures, full of dense connective tissue (sheets of fascia, ligaments, membranes, blood vessels, and more). Because of this, they are highly susceptible to fluid buildup. That means that over the course of your workout (or even prolonged sitting), blood and excess fluid will build up in your legs, especially in this area. Because your calves are so dense, they need help getting that fluid out, otherwise pressure builds and can stiffen your connective tissue. It's kind of like a sausage casing that's got too much sausage in it—at a certain point it will burst. And you better believe that this stress on your system will transfer strain down your leg into your Achilles and foot, not to mention your shins.

Unfortunately, static (still) stretching— what most people turn to—is simply not an effective remedy.

✔ SOLUTION

PUMP YOUR **CALVES**

Active calf pumping is the way to go. While it requires more effort than hanging your heel off a curb, this kind of dynamic stretching will help increase circulation through your lower legs and maintain fluidity through your calves. Added bonus: It's preventive medicine for your feet.

It's worth noting that many self-proclaimed "toe runners"—those who rely heavily on their forefoot to power their stride—are overworking their calves due to lazy glutes. If you think this might be you, make sure you Wake Up Your Butt (p. 107).

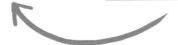

Fluidity = Ability to move with optimal power and minimal compensation

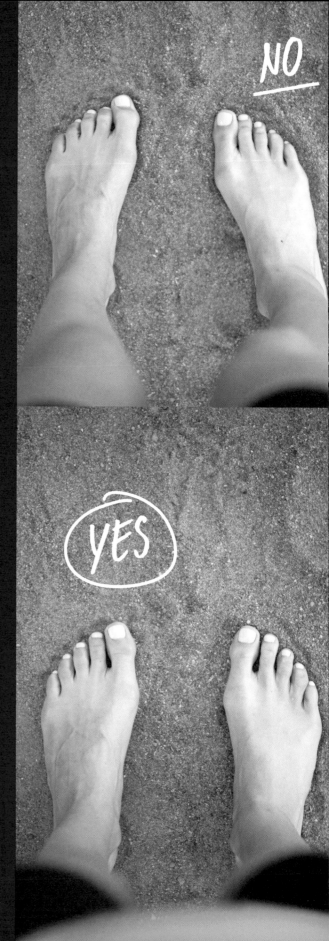

WHERE'S
YOUR WEIGHT?

Use this assessment to become more aware of how you're standing, remembering that your foot alignment has a profound impact on your entire system.

> Take your shoes off and stand as you would between reps at the gym or in line at the grocery store—don't overthink it, just stand there.

> Without shifting your weight, focus on your feet. Take note of how stable your foundation is and notice where your weight is on your feet:

Are you loading up the balls of your feet?

Are you leaning back into your heels?

Are the arches of your feet doing anything?

Are your toes gripping the floor?

Where is your center of gravity?

Once you're aware of what's going on down there, you can proactively correct toward center.

✔ CORRECT

When you **establish a balanced foundation,** your body can more readily find optimal alignment—which will help you improve your posture and biomechanics:

> Stand with your feet hip width apart— this is about two fists for most of us— stacking your knees over your ankles and your hips over your knees.

> Bend your knees slightly and close your eyes.

> Rock your weight forward toward the balls of your feet.

> Rock your weight back toward your heels.

> Rock forward and back a couple of times, then find the center and stop there.

> Rock your weight toward the outer edges of your feet and back in toward the arches of your feet a couple of times, then stop in the center.

> Lift up your toes—you'll feel your arches activate—and try to spread them out before setting them down, without gripping the floor.

> Press down strongly and evenly through your feet, keeping your arches active.

> Notice if this feels any different from how you'd casually stand.

This is what it means to establish a balanced foundation—it's not just about shifting your center of gravity, it's about aligning your joints and activating your neutral base (your feet). This is the starting point for most standing poses.

NOTICE HOW YOU'RE STANDING

HIT RESET TO BALANCE YOUR FOUNDATION

ROUTINES

- ✔ **Fix Your Feet** (p. 63)
- ✔ **Pump Your Calves** (p. 66)

BENEFITS

- ❯ Become aware of and activate your foot muscles so you can use them to full advantage
- ❯ Maintain circulation through the calf musculature to facilitate fluidity in the lower legs
- ❯ Mitigate the effects of wearing shoes all the time
- ❯ Help prevent lower leg and foot strain and compensation injuries

PRACTICE	Pre-workout/crosstraining
HOW LONG	Hold for 5–8 breaths or 10+ reps/multiple sets for movement
PROPS	Folded towel or blanket
RED FLAGS	Lower leg and foot injuries Toes sticking together or gripping the floor

FIND THE CENTER

✔ FIX YOUR **FEET**

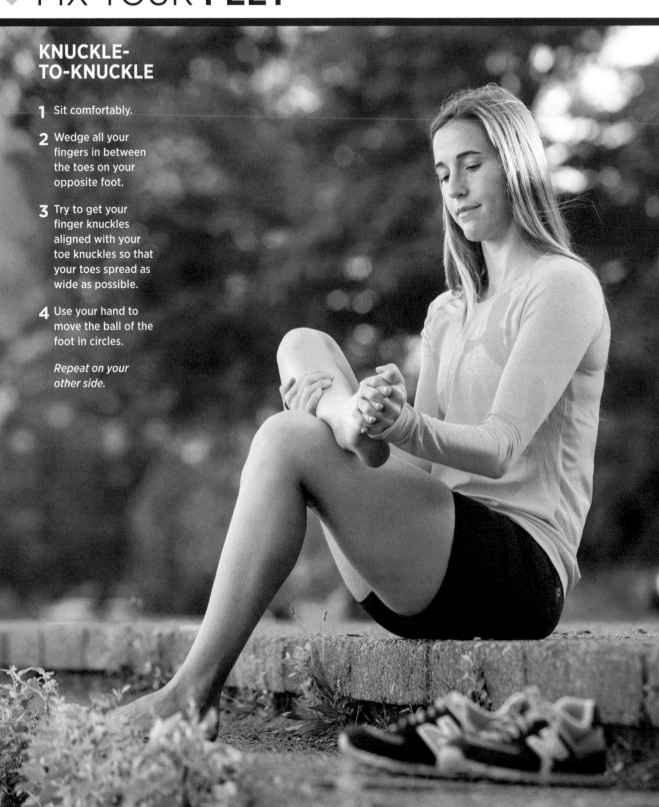

KNUCKLE-TO-KNUCKLE

1 Sit comfortably.

2 Wedge all your fingers in between the toes on your opposite foot.

3 Try to get your finger knuckles aligned with your toe knuckles so that your toes spread as wide as possible.

4 Use your hand to move the ball of the foot in circles.

Repeat on your other side.

TOE YOGA

1 Sit comfortably with your foot flat on the floor, evenly distributing pressure across the ball of your foot.

2 Lift your big toe up (keeping the other toes on the floor), and use your fingers to create resistance as you slowly push the toe down to the floor.

3 After you've done some reps like this, see if you can lift and lower your big toe independently of the rest of your toes (keeping them on the floor) without using your fingers for help—practice!

Repeat on your other side.

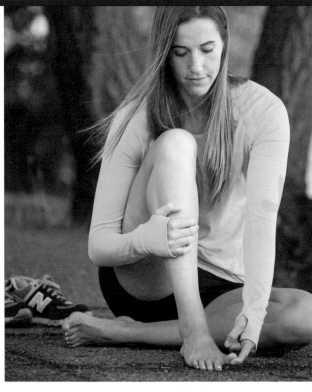

PERCH

Forward

1 From all fours, tuck your toes under. Reach back and pull your baby toes forward, even if they don't want to stay there.

2 Walk your hands forward, as if you're pushing the floor away from you.

3 Push your butt toward your heels, and push your heels back.

>> Put a folded towel or blanket under your knees for padding if needed.

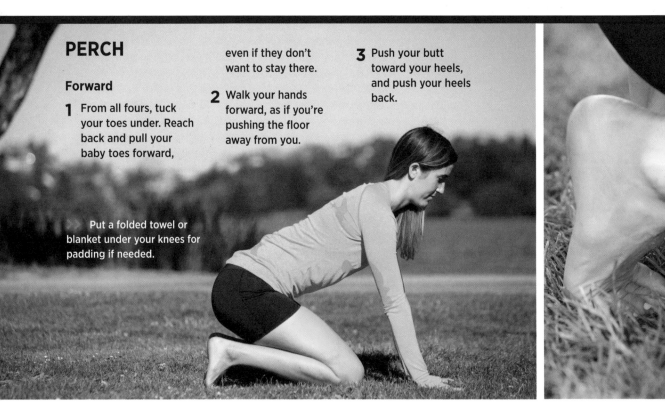

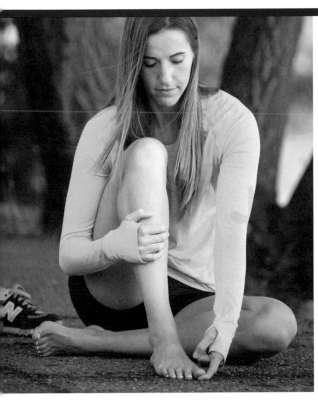
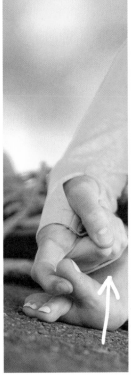
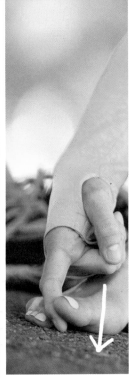

Upright

1 Walk your hands onto your thighs and sit upright, leaning your weight back slightly.

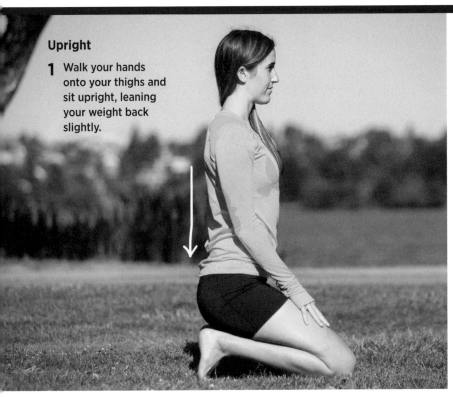
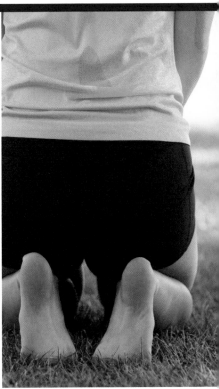

PUMP YOUR **CALVES**

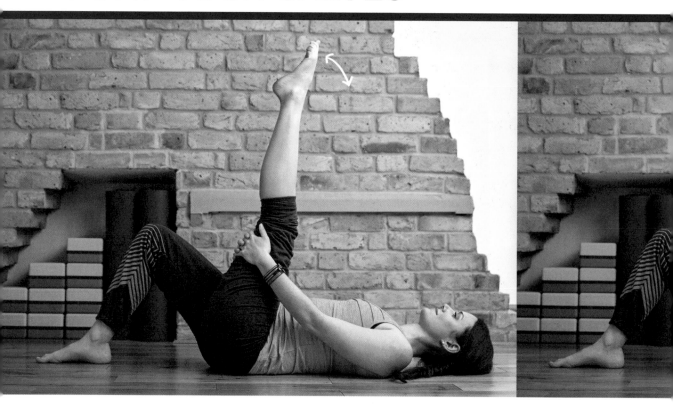

SQUAT CALF PUMP

1 Step your feet wider than hip width apart, externally rotating your thighs in your hip joints so that your legs turn away from the center of your body (your heels point in and toes point out).

2 Bend your knees deeply to come down into a squat, resting your hands on the floor between your legs.

3 Stay up higher, resting your hands on a prop for support if your knees are uncomfortable in a deep squat.

4 Lift your heels as high as you can.

5 Drop your heels toward the floor.

6 Continue …

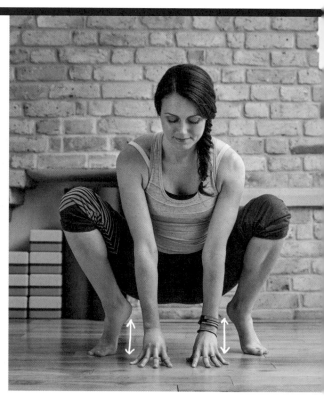

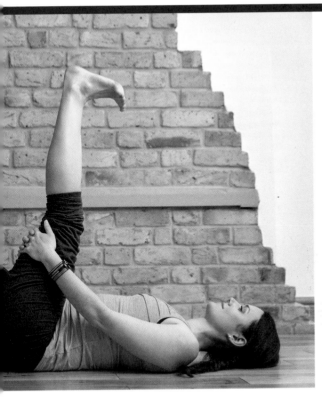

HAMMY TIME POINT & FLEX

1 Lie on your back.

2 Extend one leg toward the ceiling and interlace your fingers around your hamstrings, making a hammock for that leg to rest into.

3 Bend your other knee and put that foot on the floor, helping you to maintain a neutral spine.

4 Point your lifted-leg foot.

5 Flex your lifted-leg foot.

6 Continue …

Repeat on your other side.

>> Your arms should be straight, shoulders and head on the floor—bend your lifted-leg knee as much as needed to make that happen.

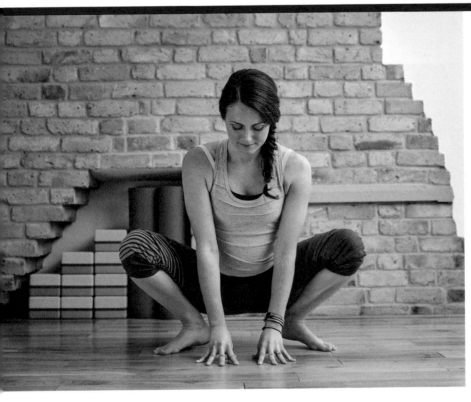

ALL FOURS CALF PUMP

Straight leg

1 From all fours, straighten one leg behind you, tucking your toes under on the floor.

2 Keeping your hips level, rock your weight forward and back, as if you're doing standing heel lifts on that leg.

3 Continue for 10 reps, then come to stillness as you press back strongly through your heel.

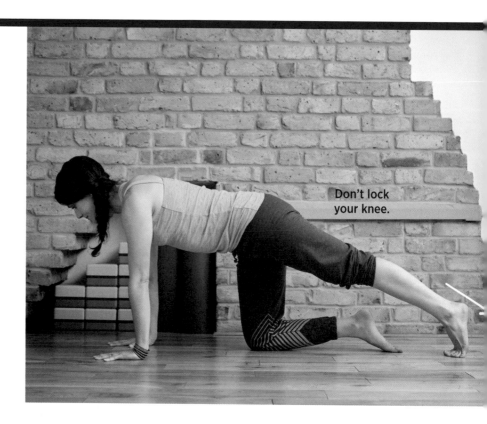

Don't lock your knee.

Bent knee

1 Continue to press back through your heel and bend your extended leg knee more.

2 Straighten the leg without locking the knee.

3 Continue …

Repeat on your other side.

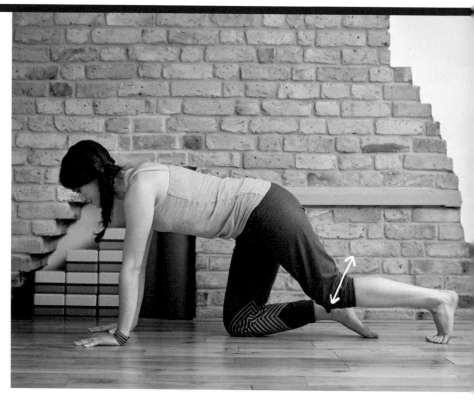

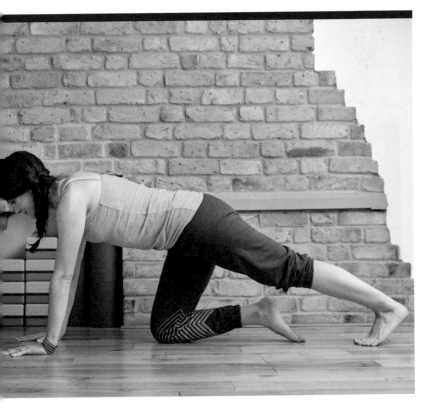

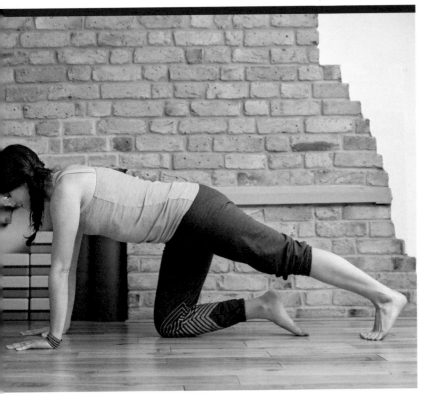

FAQ Why work with both a straight leg and a bent knee in calf stretching?

Ever notice how it feels a bit different when you stretch your calves with knees bent compared to straight legs? That's because there's more musculature in your calves than just the larger surface-layer muscles soleus and gastroc. When your legs are straight, you hit those big surface guys.

When you add a bend in your knees, you take the slack off the surface muscles—the influence of gastroc is eliminated altogether because it crosses the knee—and can address the smaller, deeper muscles of the calf that are responsible for pointing and flexing the foot. It's these deeper muscles that are much more likely to be ignored and in turn get sticky and create issues. The difference might feel more subtle, but any pumping movement with a bent knee will help you increase circulation and tone in those muscles.

HEEL LIFTS

1 Establish a balanced foundation (p. 61).

2 Lift your heels high.

3 Lower your heels to hover above the floor.

4 Do a set with your legs straight (but knees not locked), then do a set with bent knees.

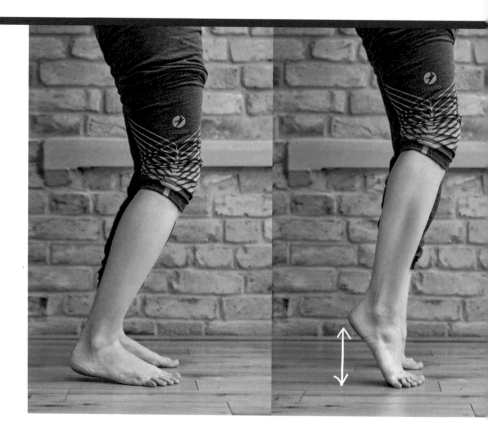

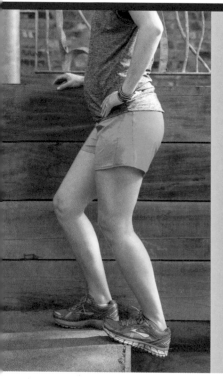

BONUS Take it to the steps

This exercise is the same as Heel Lifts, but you stand with the balls of your feet on the edge of a step so that your heels can drop farther. This is a fantastic eccentric strengthener—it causes tissues to contract while they're lengthening—and is really helpful for preventing calf and Achilles issues.

GAME
PLAN

! When I stand casually, my weight tends to shift:

✔ Even though I wear shoes all the time, I'll keep my feet awake by:

#hitreset

✔ What are you doing to balance your foundation today?

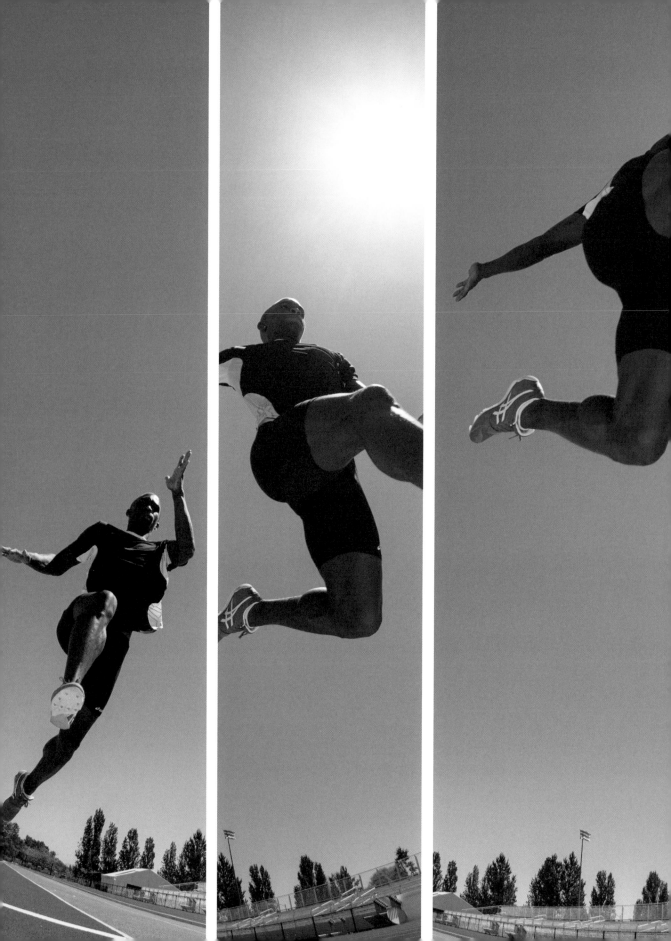

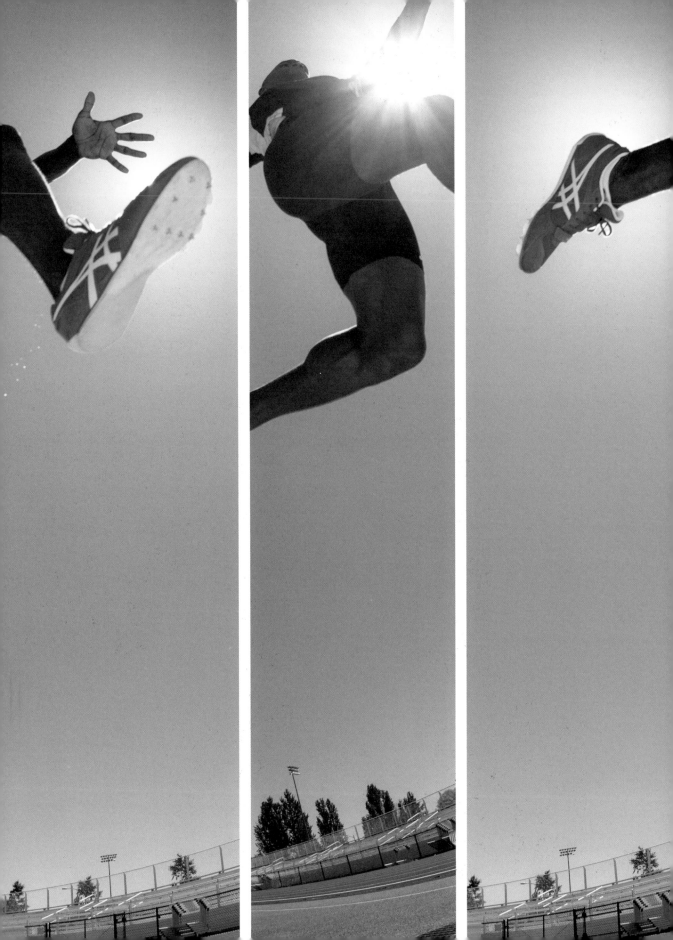

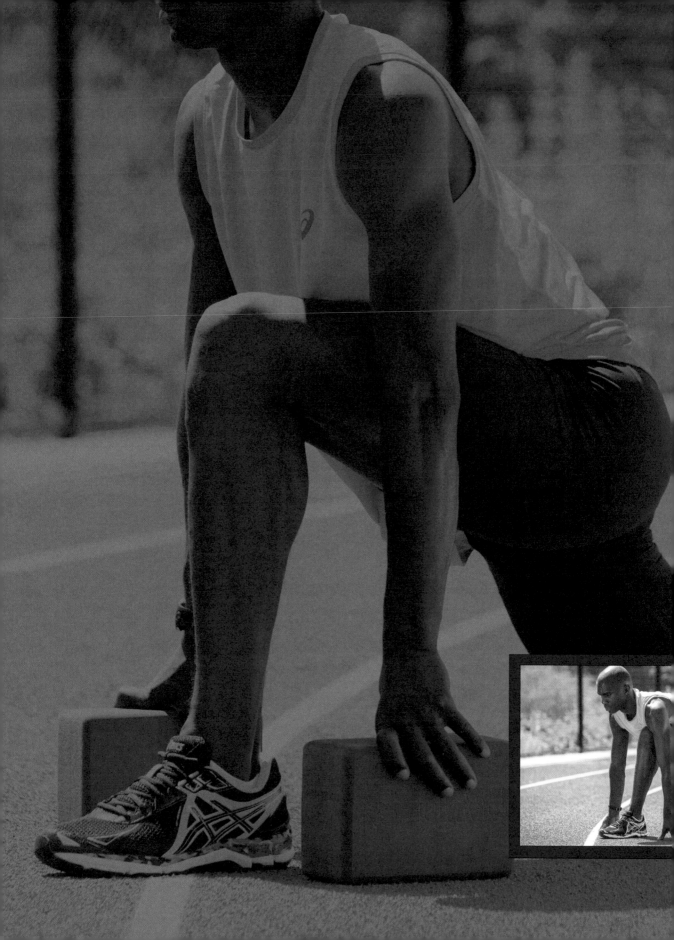

SAVE *YOUR* KNEES

Knees are particularly susceptible to wear and tear because they're inherently unstable. You've got muscles that move them—however, these muscles don't do a very good job of stabilizing them, which is problematic because a balance of mobility and stability is critical for optimal function. Ultimately, the health of your knees depends largely on good joint alignment and balanced strength and flexibility in the hips. Maintenance in these areas will take some work, but it's worth the effort.

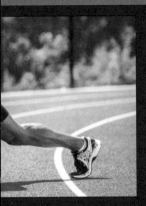
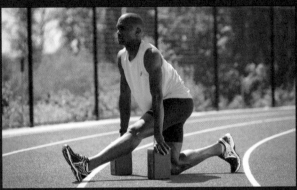
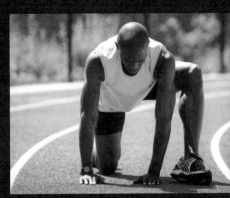

Unstable knees are injury-prone

Muscles are designed to both move joints and keep them stable. Ligaments, tendons, and other soft tissue are there to attach things and help out. Because the knee joint relies heavily on ligaments for stability, it is particularly vulnerable to injury. This becomes super-risky when you start racing around without paying attention to joint alignment. For example, if your knees aren't tracking forward over your ankles, they're not aligned optimally and as a result will be less stable, which increases your injury risk. The same is true if you're a chronic knee-locker—your joints are unstable, and you will continue to increase that instability (and become more injury-prone) over time.

✔ SOLUTION
MITIGATE **BOOTY LOCK**

Initiate movement from your hips, where you have more strength and stability to draw upon. Maintaining a healthy range of motion in your hips will make this possible and help prevent knee injuries. It's not a quick fix—it takes time to unlock your hips, and once you've gained full range of motion, it's use it or lose it! You need to commit to ongoing maintenance, regardless of your sport or goals. Head to the Mitigate Booty Lock routine (p. 123) for more practice and inspiration.

✔ SOLUTION
ALIGN YOUR **STRIDE**

Luckily, whether you realize it or not, the basic lunge is one of your most fundamental movements in sports and in life—it's basically what you do when you walk and run—and mastering it is key for preventing injuries. Practicing variations on this classic pose will help you create optimal alignment, stabilize your joints, and increase fluidity in the surrounding muscles so that they don't pull your knees out of their happy medium.

! PROBLEM

Stiff hips cause knee strain

Lacking range of motion in the hips will place excess strain on your knees. Here's what happens: When your thighbone can't move freely in your hip joint, the next point of least resistance is your knees. In other words, the movement you're trying to make will place excess strain on your knee and ultimately force your knee joint to move in ways it's not designed to in order to compensate for your hip's inability to achieve optimal function. Ouch.

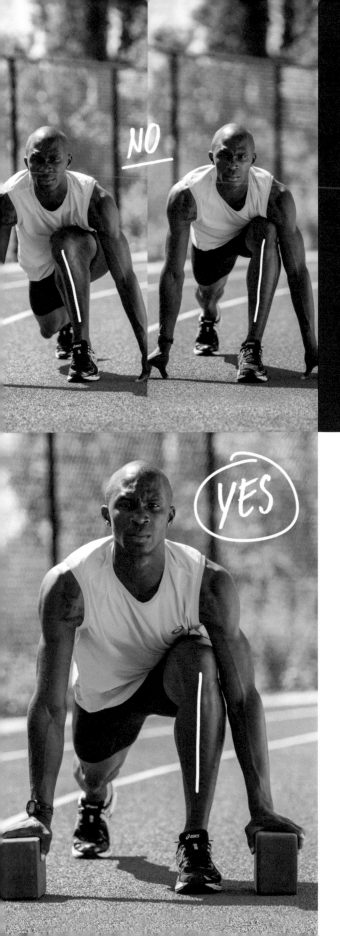

HOW'S YOUR **FORM?**

Use this assessment to gain clarity about your biomechanics. Remember, it's very likely that whatever happens when you lunge is also happening when you walk and run. Try it:

> Step one leg back into a lunge. Once you feel relatively stable, notice your alignment tendencies, especially what's going on in your hip, knee, ankle, and foot:

Is your knee collapsing toward the center?

Is your knee flopping to the side?

Is your knee over your ankle?

Is the inner arch of your foot collapsed?

Are your toes gripping the floor?

✔ CORRECT

Here are some key alignment points to ensure solid form when you practice lunge variations, whether on your yoga mat, in the weight room, or during drills on the track.

> Put blocks under your hands if you're straining to reach the floor.

> Press down evenly through your front foot—don't grip the floor with your toes.

> Make sure your knee is tracking over your ankle, not flopping to the right or left.

> If it's hard to get your foot all the way under your knee, grab that ankle with your hand and pull the foot all the way up there.

> Gently hug the knees toward each other—maintain the integrity of the lunge by keeping everything stable rather than just hanging out (and letting your hips sag toward the floor).

HIT RESET
TO SAVE YOUR KNEES

ROUTINES
✔ **Align Your Stride** (p. 79)
✔ **Mitigate Booty Lock** (p. 123)

BENEFITS
> Increase hip and hamstring flexibility
> Improve knee, hip, and ankle stability
> Improve awareness of proper alignment
> Help prevent knee strain and compensation injuries

PRACTICE	Pre-workout/crosstraining (Align Your Stride) Post-workout/recovery (Mitigate Booty Lock)
HOW LONG	Hold for 5–8 breaths or 10+ reps/multiple sets for movement
PROPS	Folded towel or blanket and blocks or water bottles
RED FLAGS	Poor foot alignment Knee tracking issues Spinal compensation Knee injuries

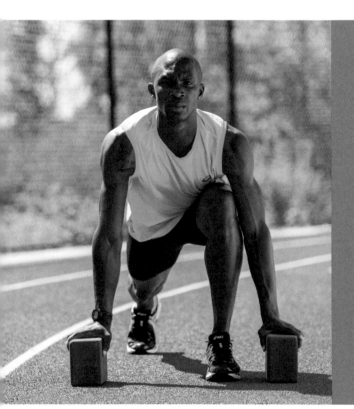

TECHNIQUE
Bring the floor to you

The floor isn't the goal—there's nothing down there for you! There's no point in straining to reach the floor, because your body will compensate in all kinds of funky ways when you force it. If you can't easily reach the floor, bring the floor up to meet you using blocks, water bottles, or whatever props you have handy.

PROPS TO THOSE WHO USE BLOCKS

ALIGN **YOUR STRIDE**

Do this routine first on one side, then pause to feel the difference before repeating the full routine on your other side.

LOW LUNGE

1 Step one leg back into a lunge and lower your back knee to the floor—pad your knee if needed.

2 Frame your front foot with your hands— place props beneath your hands if needed.

3 Pick up your back knee, pull it back another inch, and return the knee to the floor, encouraging your stride to lengthen.

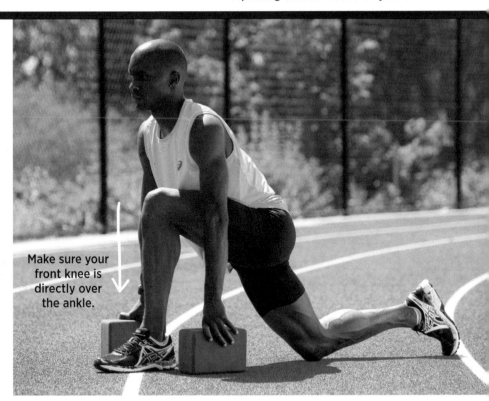

Make sure your front knee is directly over the ankle.

RUNNER'S LUNGE

1 Step one leg back into a lunge and frame your front foot with your hands.

2 Keep your back knee lifted and engage that leg to make it as straight and active as possible.

3 Keep your spine as neutral as possible, rather than side bending—make sure your front-leg-side waist hasn't shortened.

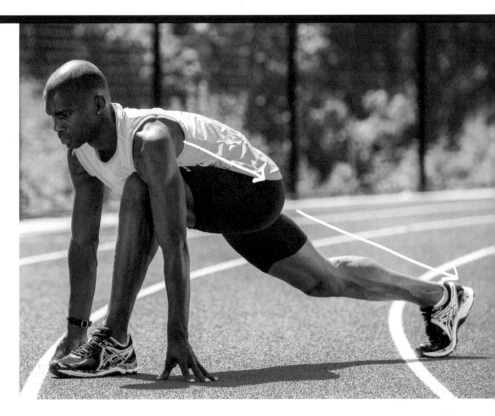

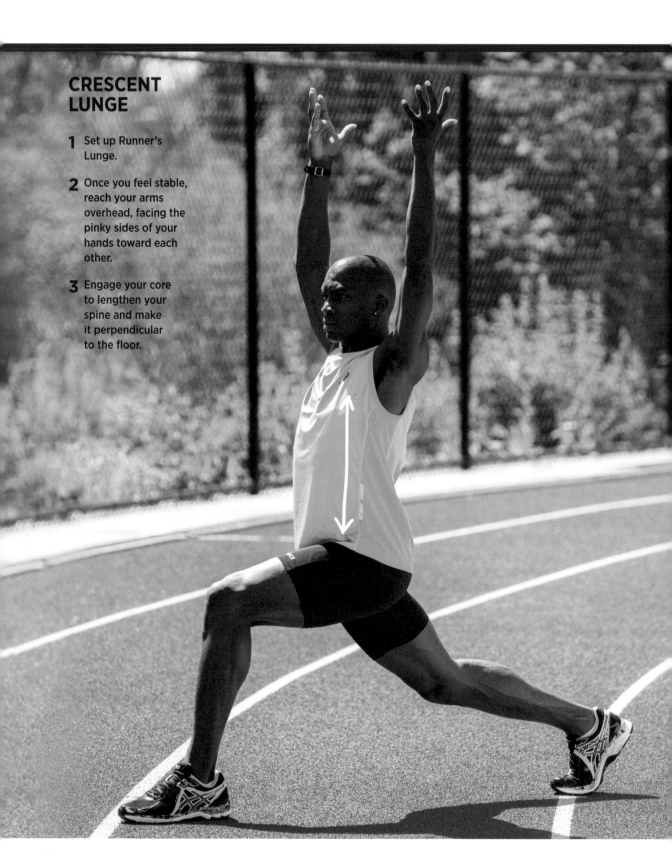

CRESCENT LUNGE

1 Set up Runner's Lunge.

2 Once you feel stable, reach your arms overhead, facing the pinky sides of your hands toward each other.

3 Engage your core to lengthen your spine and make it perpendicular to the floor.

HALF SPLIT

1 From Low Lunge, straighten your front leg as much as you can without locking the knee, walking your hands back as much as necessary.

2 Flex your front foot so that the toes point up.

3 Dig your front heel into the floor and move the hip of that leg back, away from your shoulder on that side—it's kind of like your heel is stuck but you're trying to drag it toward you.

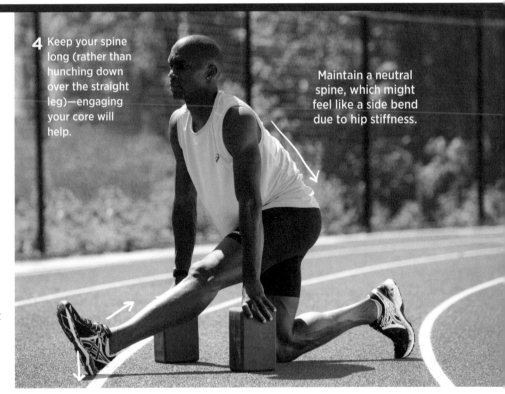

4 Keep your spine long (rather than hunching down over the straight leg)—engaging your core will help.

Maintain a neutral spine, which might feel like a side bend due to hip stiffness.

HALF SPLIT ROTATION

1 From Half Split, turn out your thigh in your hip joint.

2 Turn in your thigh in your hip joint.

3 Continue, feeling the natural stopping point, aka the end of your hip range of motion, and then rotate back in the other direction, using the muscles in your hip to steer the movement rather than just turning your foot.

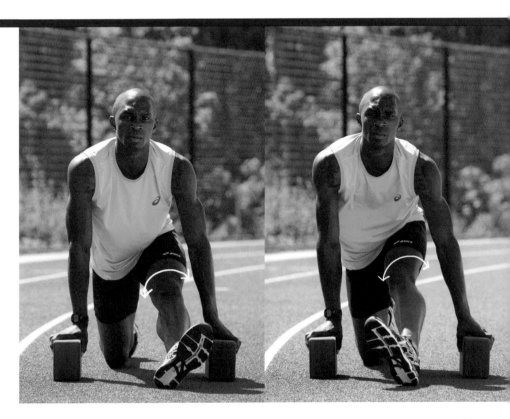

LUNGE FLOW

1 From Low Lunge, lengthen your front leg into Half Split, flexing your foot and keeping your spine long.

2 Continue, moving forward and backward.

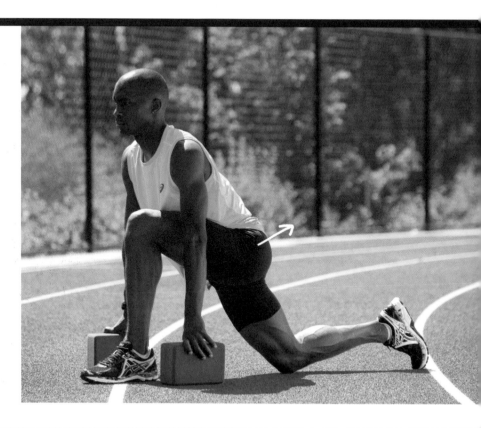

LIZARD

1 From Low Lunge, move your front foot over to the side, away from the center of your body, and turn out your thigh.

2 Rest your hands on the floor beneath your chest.

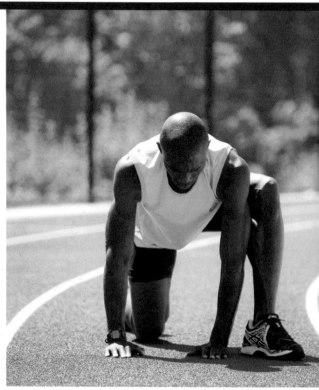

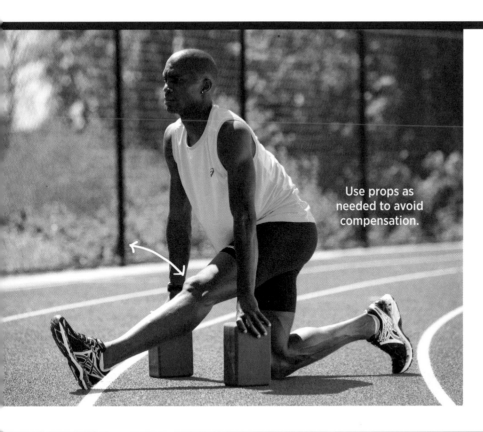

Use props as needed to avoid compensation.

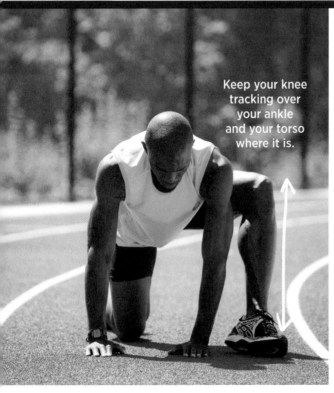

Keep your knee tracking over your ankle and your torso where it is.

LIZARD FLOW

1 From Lizard, rock toward the outside edge of your front foot—your leg will move a few inches away from your body.

2 Bring your leg back in toward your body, returning the foot flat to the floor.

3 Continue, steering from your hip so that your knee/ankle/foot are all tracking together, in alignment.

Pause and feel the difference between sides before doing the routine on your other side, beginning with Low Lunge.

GAME
PLAN

! My knees are prone to compensate when:

! When I lunge, my main misalignment is:

✔ I'll take time to align my stride when:

#hitreset

✔ What are you doing to save your knees today?

LOCKED JOINTS
ARE UNSTABLE—
UNLOCK
YOUR KNEES!

DO THE
**LITTLE
THINGS**

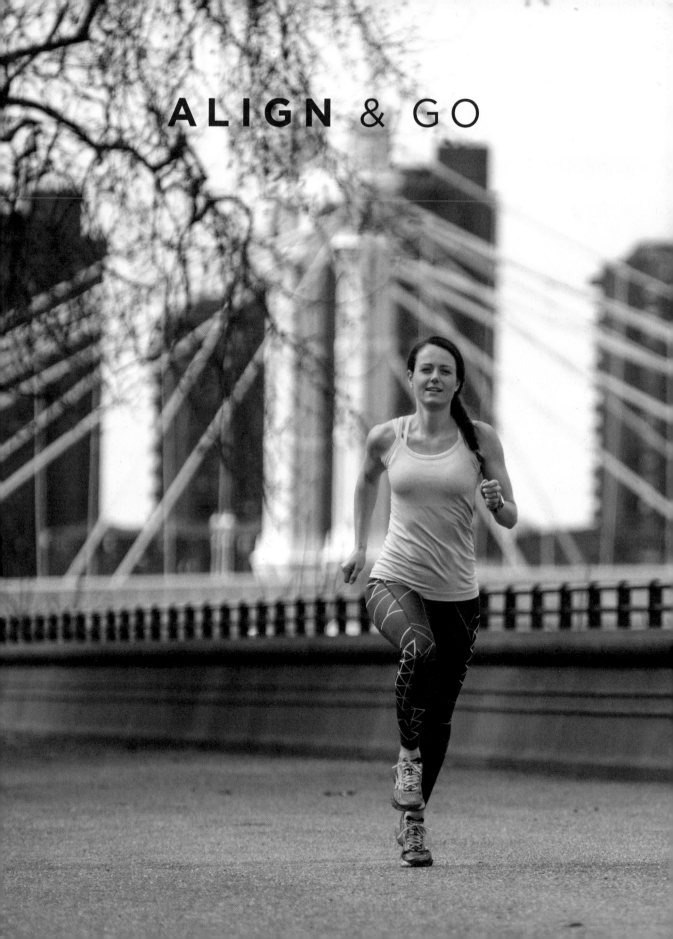

ALIGN & GO

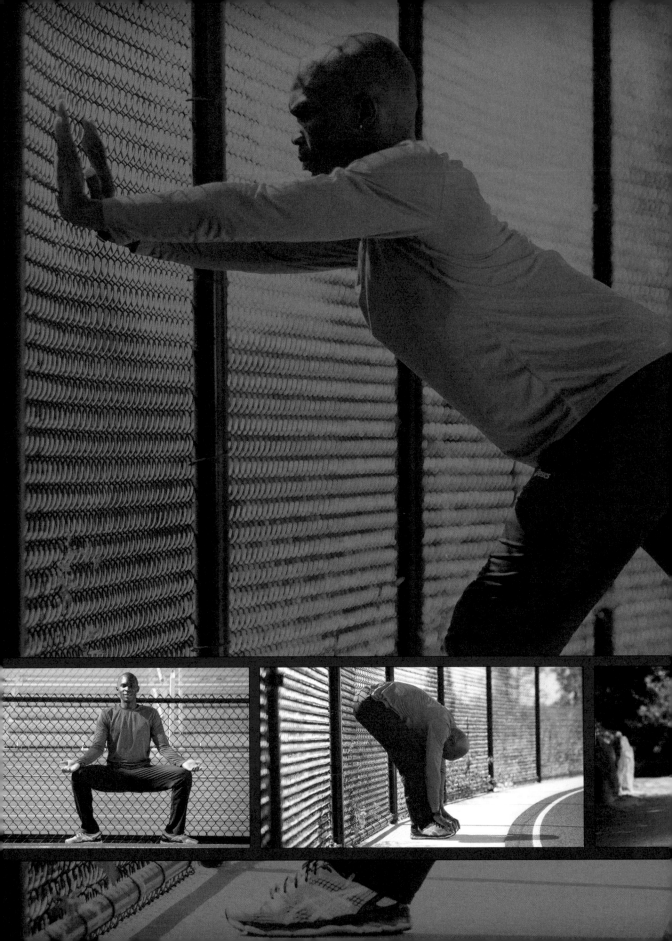

UNSTIFFEN *YOUR*
HAMSTRINGS

People don't pay much attention to their hamstrings, other than to moan about how stiff they are. The fact is we could all use a little hammy time.

This muscle group is prone to dysfunction because we sit so much. As a result, the hamstrings become tight, dry, and stuck together. Similarly, if you fail to stretch after your workout, your hamstrings will become—you guessed it—tight, dry, and stuck together. You'll be shuffling around like a zombie. And, despite your best attempts, common tactics such as locking your knees as you struggle to reach the floor or throwing your leg up and yanking on those tissues with a strap are more likely to injure your hamstrings than unstiffen them.

The culprits behind most hamstring issues go hand-in-hand …

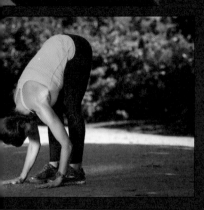

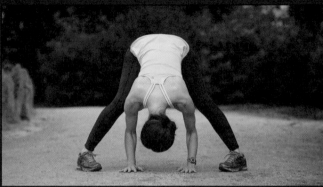

Stiff hamstrings lack fluidity

Tight, dry, stuck-together muscles can't move fluidly—or optimally.

This is a matter of circulation. Most of us sit on our hamstrings all day, which isn't conducive to good circulation. Then, when you hop out of your chair to walk home, go for a run, or chase your kids around, those stiff hammies cannot access their full range of motion and they become more injury-prone.

YOUR HAMSTRINGS SHOULD BE LIKE RUBBER BANDS, NOT GUITAR STRINGS

! PROBLEM

Poor awareness leads to strain

Optimal hamstring flexibility isn't about being able to touch your toes. It's about maintaining fluidity and aligning your body properly so that you can effectively access a full range of motion safely. Basic awareness is key for ensuring you are stretching, not straining, which can lead to pulled muscles. If your alignment is poor, you are likely to sprain your ligaments whether you are bending over to pick up a weight or your groceries. These soft connective tissues don't bounce back like muscles do—once stretched out, they stay that way, which leads to instability and injury.

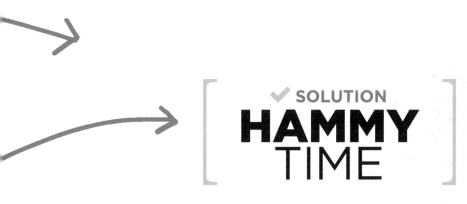

✔ **SOLUTION**
HAMMY
TIME

While many people turn to yoga to improve hamstring flexibility, those who dive in too fast often end up injuring themselves on the mat. The best way to stay safe while unstiffening your hamstrings is to slow down and pay attention. If you go too hard too fast, your muscles will fight back.

Ultimately, it's a combination of active and passive stretching that will increase and sustain your flexibility and range of motion—this is the goal. Active stretches are dynamic stretches that increase blood flow while lengthening the tissue, and they allow you to increase the intensity on your own. These poses are most effective pre-workout, although they can be done post-workout as well. Passive stretches are more restorative stretches that rely on external forces such as gravity or props to ease the muscles that have worked hard for you by softening their surrounding connective tissues, so you'll get the most benefit if you do them post-workout. As you increase your fluidity and awareness, your hamstring flexibility and the range of motion in your hips will improve significantly.

Hammy time =
Active + Passive hamstring stretching

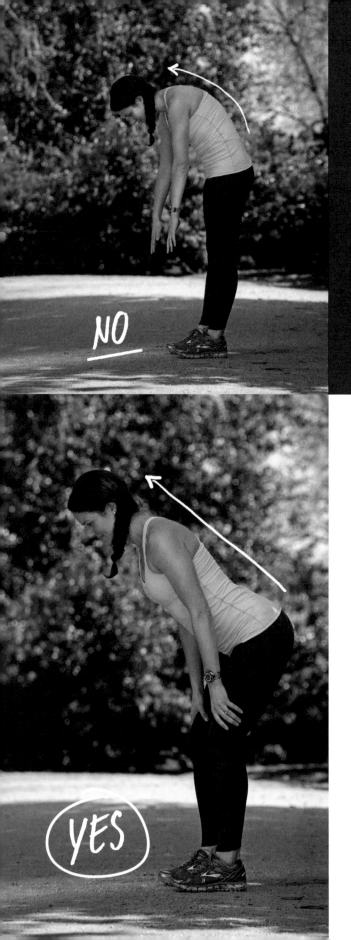

NO

YES

! **SELF-TEST**

WHAT'S GOING ON
BACK THERE?

> Stand in profile in front of a full-length mirror.

> Bend down to touch your toes as you usually would, without thinking much about it.

> Stay down there and turn your head so that you can see what you look like— in particular, notice your knees, spine, and butt.

✔ CORRECT

A floppy forward fold will eventually strain your ligaments. Set yourself up for hammy time success:

> Establish a balanced foundation (p. 61). Bring your feet hip width apart and parallel, evenly distributing your weight across both feet.

> Bend your knees—a lot! Imagine you're pushing your shins forward while keeping your hips where they are—it will feel a bit like you're sticking your butt out.

> Lengthen your spine. Stand tall before you ever begin the stretch, relaxing your shoulders so that your posture is optimized for the pose.

> Keep your spine long as you descend into your forward fold. Slowly walk your hands down your legs, lengthening your torso as you go. If you feel your spine start to round, stop where you are, resting your hands on your legs or props for support.

HIT RESET TO UNSTIFFEN YOUR HAMSTRINGS

ROUTINES

✔ **Find Fluidity** (p. 92)

✔ **Restore Your Range** (p. 98)

BENEFITS

> Increase fluidity in your hamstrings so you can use them to full advantage

> Improve awareness of how to stretch effectively

> Prevent hamstring and back strain and the resulting compensation injuries

PRACTICE	Pre-workout/recovery (Find Fluidity) Post-workout (Find Fluidity, Restore Your Range)
HOW LONG	Hold for 5–8 breaths or 10+ reps/multiple sets for movement
PROPS	Blocks
RED FLAGS	Knee locking Spinal compensation via rounding forward Straining to reach the floor Hamstring and back injuries

FAQ Why am I flopping forward?

Hamstring stretching isn't a race to touch your toes. When the hammies are stiff—which is usually the reality for athletes—they pull the pelvis away from neutral. Also known as posterior tilt, this looks a bit like your tail is tucked or you have a flat butt. When you begin from this tilted position, it's nearly impossible to stretch the belly of the hamstring muscles (the meatiest part, right in the middle) because the low back is so rounded, or flexed. Instead, the stretch just turns into this hunchy, floppy thing. By bending your knees and keeping your pelvis neutral, you can help protect your ligaments and direct the stretch into the bellies of your hamstrings—where it's meant to be.

✔ FIND **FLUIDITY**

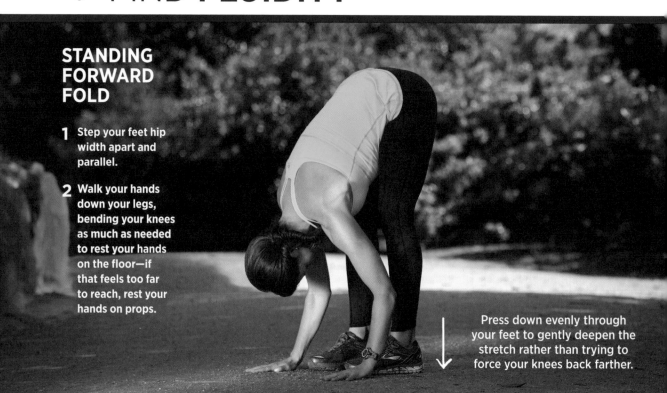

STANDING FORWARD FOLD

1 Step your feet hip width apart and parallel.

2 Walk your hands down your legs, bending your knees as much as needed to rest your hands on the floor—if that feels too far to reach, rest your hands on props.

Press down evenly through your feet to gently deepen the stretch rather than trying to force your knees back farther.

TECHNIQUE

Bend & stretch

The last thing you want to do is to yank on angry hammies. When you first come into a forward fold, give your knees a generous bend and then bend and stretch your legs at least 10 times—this should be a small movement. This is key because it will help you address the issues of fluidity and awareness by:

> Slowly drawing the circulation into the area you want to stretch (your hamstrings).

> Increasing your awareness of where you want to feel the stretch—in the muscle bellies rather than other soft tissue such as the backs of your knees or where your hamstrings attach to your pelvis.

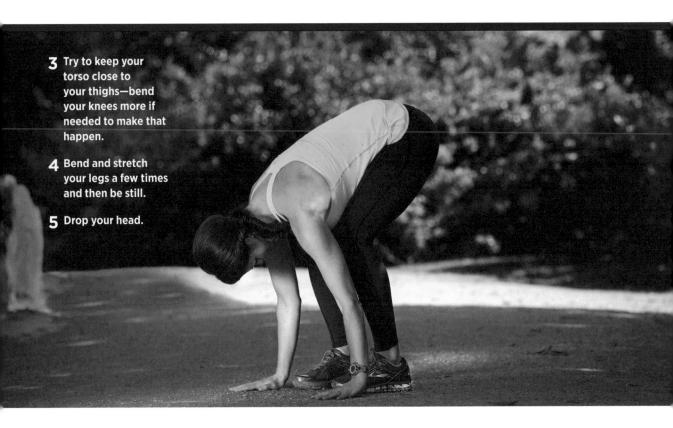

3 Try to keep your torso close to your thighs—bend your knees more if needed to make that happen.

4 Bend and stretch your legs a few times and then be still.

5 Drop your head.

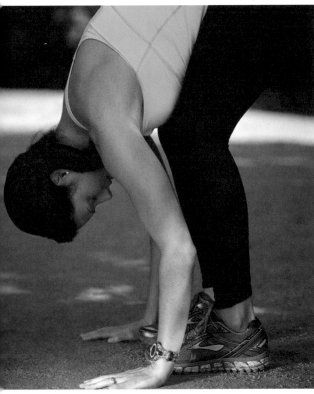

>> When you get all the way down into your fold, a good way to tell if your spine is still long is to try to keep your torso close to your thighs. You might find that you have to bend your knees more to make this happen.

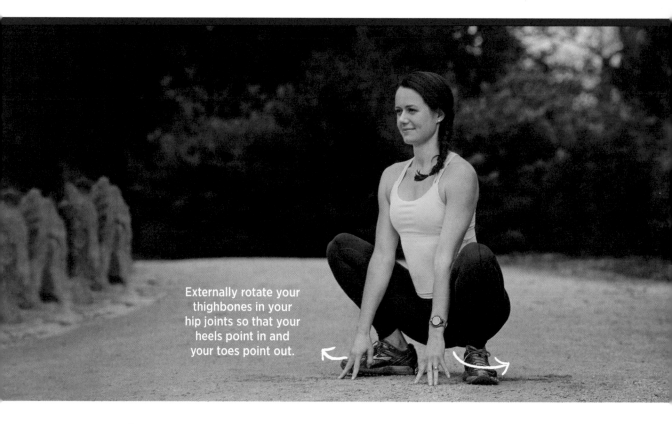

Externally rotate your thighbones in your hip joints so that your heels point in and your toes point out.

SQUAT/ FORWARD FOLD FLOW

1 Come into a Standing Forward Fold with your feet a bit wider than hip width apart.

2 Turn out your thighs and bend your knees deeply to come down into a squat, keeping your weight back toward your heels—stay as high as needed to keep your heels down, and take the feet wider apart if needed.

3 Rest your hands on the floor in front of you, put your forearms on your quads, or bring your elbows to your inner thighs and join your palms in front of your chest.

4 Pivot on your heels as you straighten your legs and rotate your thighs back to neutral, returning to your Standing Forward Fold.

5 Slowly flow back and forth between Squat and Forward Fold.

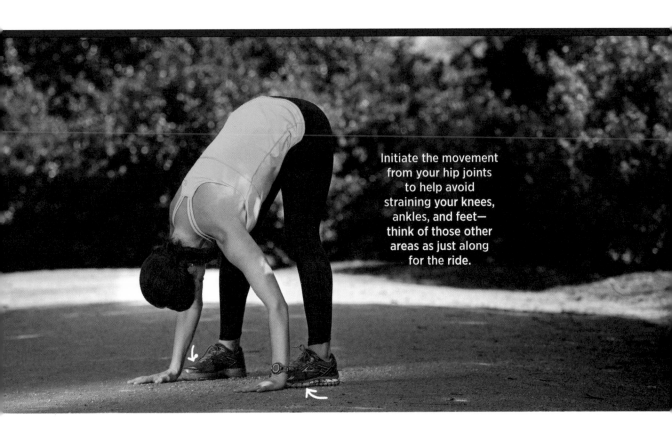

Initiate the movement from your hip joints to help avoid straining your knees, ankles, and feet— think of those other areas as just along for the ride.

STOP STRUGGLING TO REACH YOUR TOES— STRETCH WHERE YOU ARE NOW

Stretch smarter

Technically, you've got three hammies. They include your outer hamstring (biceps femoris) and a pair of inner hamstrings (semitendinosus and semimembranosus). However, there is an additional muscle that, although it is your most powerful adductor, also acts kind of like a hamstring: Meet adductor magnus. The name is worth remembering because although people usually think hamstrings are causing their attachment-point pain, adductor magnus is a common culprit.

This is important because the "hamstring" injuries that happen in yoga often involve your adductor magnus. Given it is usually the angriest of the hammy group, you'll want to give it more slack when you first get into your forward folding practice—this is best accomplished via internal rotation, aka turning your thighs in toward each other so that your feet are slightly pigeon-toed. It's a subtle adjustment that makes a big difference. Plus, because the fibers of the aforementioned muscles extend in different directions, approaching your folding in this way will provide a more comprehensive stretch to the muscle group.

STANDING STRADDLE FORWARD FOLD

Internal rotation

1 Step your feet wide apart and turn in your thighs.

2 Walk your hands down your legs, bending your knees as much as needed to rest your hands on the floor—if that feels too far to reach, rest your hands on a block or other prop.

3 Try to keep your torso close to your thighs—bend your knees more if needed to make that happen.

4 Bend and stretch your legs a few times and then be still.

5 Press down evenly through your feet to gently deepen the stretch rather than trying to force your knees back more.

Neutral

1 From your internally rotated fold, pivot on your heels to return your thighs to neutral/feet parallel.

2 Evenly distribute your weight across your feet and continue to press down evenly through your feet.

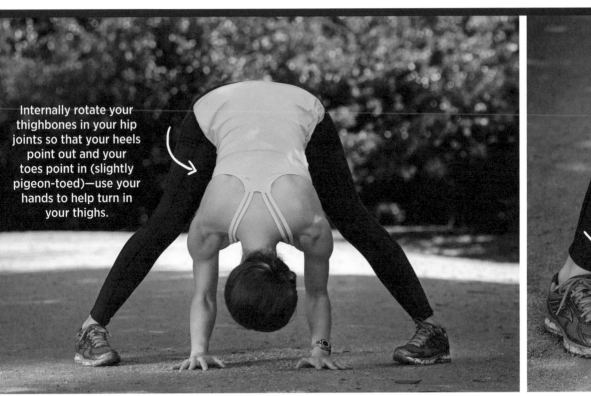

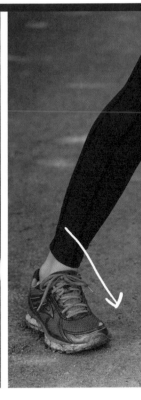

Internally rotate your thighbones in your hip joints so that your heels point out and your toes point in (slightly pigeon-toed)—use your hands to help turn in your thighs.

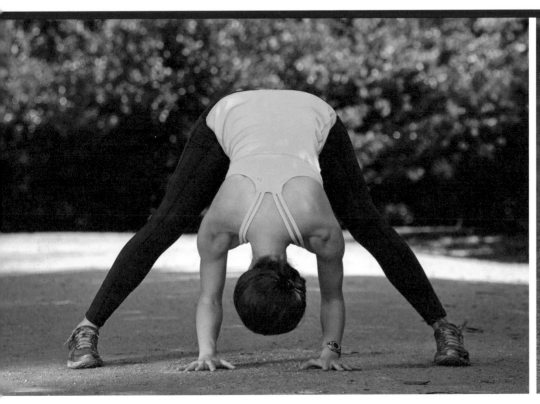

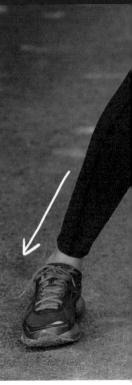

FORWARD FOLD AT THE WALL

1 Stand up and lean into the wall with your feet hip width apart and parallel, a foot or two away from the wall.

2 Keeping your knees bent, fold forward and walk your hands down your legs.

3 Lean back into the wall—if it feels hard or like you can't lean back, bring your feet a bit farther away from the wall.

4 Rest your hands wherever they land, or on props, if needed.

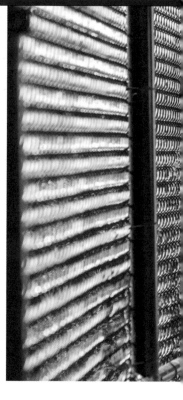

CROSSED-LEG FORWARD FOLD AT THE WALL

1 From Forward Fold at the Wall, cross one leg over the other.

2 Keep both knees bent slightly and both feet flexed so there's no torque on your ankles.

3 Keep leaning back, keeping your hips level and butt cheeks pressing evenly against the wall while you feel the support behind you.

4 Rest your hands wherever they land, or on props, if needed.

Repeat on your other side.

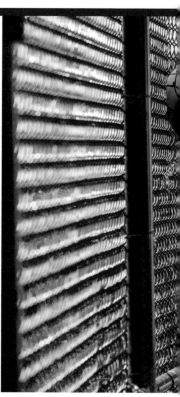

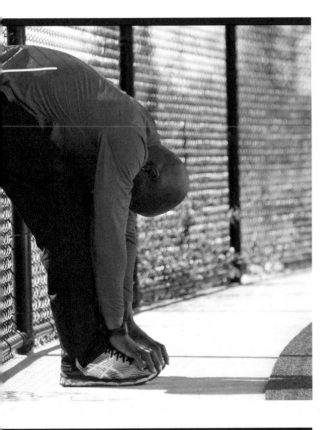

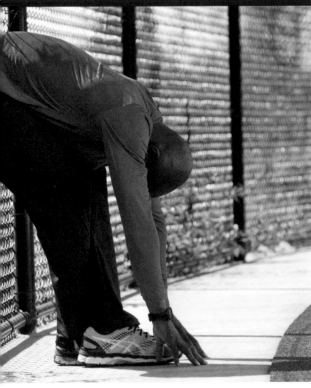

Take it to the wall

The truth is, hammy time can be tough, especially when you're tired post-workout. The good news is that there is a path of less resistance. By using a wall, fence, beam, or any sturdy surface for support, you can eliminate most of the work from the pose and really focus on the stretch rather than on trying to balance yourself. This also frees up more head space to examine your alignment—you can check that your knees aren't locking and your spine isn't rounding because you won't be working so hard to support the pose on your own.

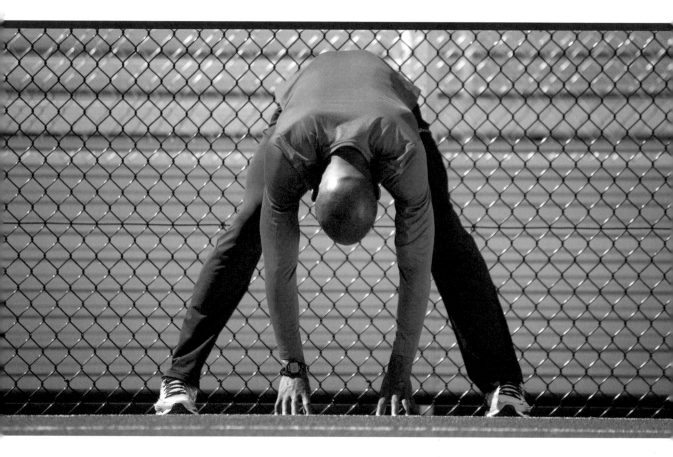

WIDE FORWARD FOLD AT THE WALL

1 Stand up and lean into the wall with your feet much wider than hip width apart and parallel, a foot or two away from the wall.

2 Keeping your knees bent, fold forward and walk your hands down your legs.

3 Lean back into the wall—if it feels hard or like you can't lean back, bring your feet a bit farther away from the wall.

4 Rest your hands wherever they land, or on props, if needed.

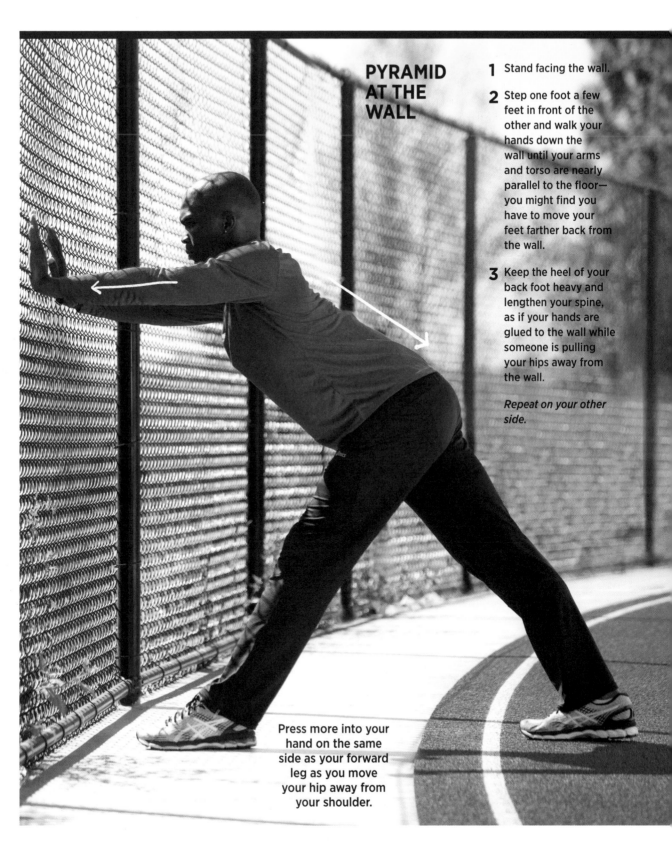

PYRAMID AT THE WALL

1 Stand facing the wall.

2 Step one foot a few feet in front of the other and walk your hands down the wall until your arms and torso are nearly parallel to the floor—you might find you have to move your feet farther back from the wall.

3 Keep the heel of your back foot heavy and lengthen your spine, as if your hands are glued to the wall while someone is pulling your hips away from the wall.

Repeat on your other side.

Press more into your hand on the same side as your forward leg as you move your hip away from your shoulder.

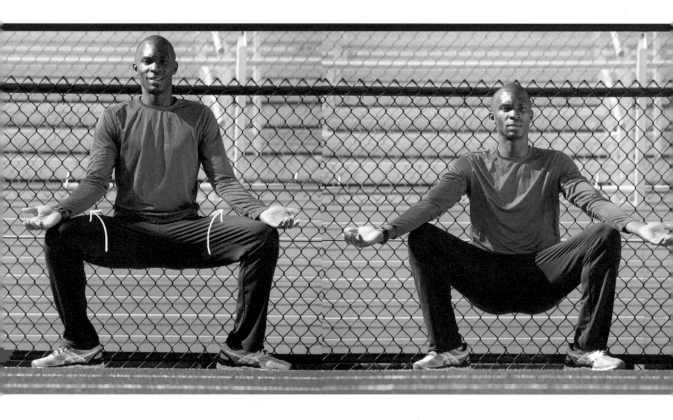

> **❝** *The brain learns as you give it new information about what the body is capable of. That 'shaking' is the recalibration of the filters between your body and your brain."*
>
> —RICHELLE RICARD, THE YOGA ENGINEER

FAQ Why am I shaking?

If you start experiencing your own personal earthquake while trying to stretch your hammies (or hold any pose, for that matter), it's a pretty good sign you've taken things too far. That said, trembles and shakes are often the result of placing an unfamiliar demand on a muscle. It makes sense: If you never stretch, your body is going to be a little confused when you try to remind it how to be flexible.

More specifically, this shaking indicates confusion in your brain, because the brain's perception governs your experience. That means the brain believes the muscle is only a certain length based on your habitual use of it. So when you take that muscle beyond its usual length, your brain shouts out, "Code red!" because you've just created a discrepancy between what is familiar and what is possible. Despite the discomfort of trying something new—like working on your flexibility—you can indeed retrain your mind and your muscles. So embrace a little shake, but make sure that you're not trembling so hard that it's causing your body undue stress.

SQUAT AT THE WALL

1 Stand up and lean into the wall with your feet wider than hip width apart.

2 Turn out your thighs and bend your knees—tracking them over the ankles—to come into a deep squat.

3 Keep leaning back into the wall, and either rest your forearms on your quads or bring your elbows to your inner thighs and join your palms in front of your chest.

4 Try to get your whole back onto the wall, even the back of your head.

5 Lift up all of your toes so you really feel your weight moving back into the heels.

>> Externally rotate your thighbones in your hip joints so that your heels point in and your toes point out.

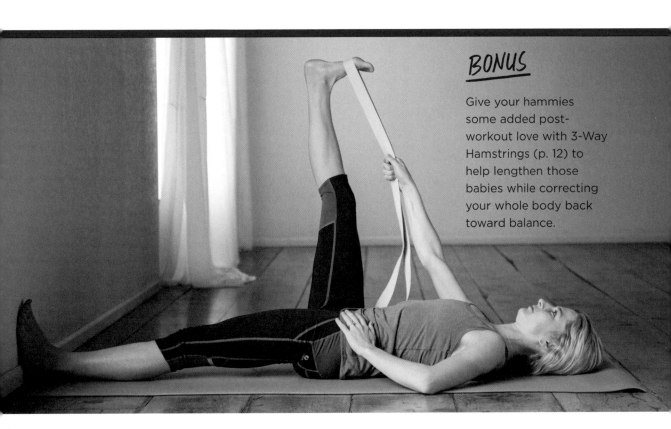

BONUS

Give your hammies some added post-workout love with 3-Way Hamstrings (p. 12) to help lengthen those babies while correcting your whole body back toward balance.

GAME
PLAN

! My hamstrings feel stiffest when:

! This impedes my sports movement/ performance by:

✓ I'll find a balance of active (Find Fluidity) and passive (Restore Your Range) hammy time by:

#hitreset

✓ What are you doing to unstiffen your hamstrings today?

FOLD, THEN BEND AND STRETCH

DO THE
**LITTLE
THINGS**

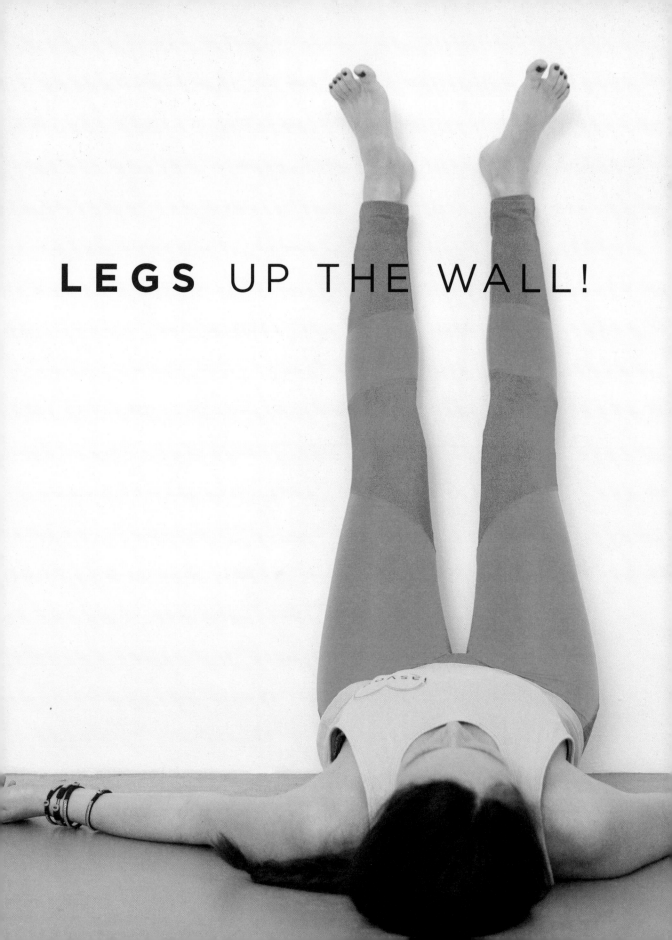

LEGS UP THE WALL!

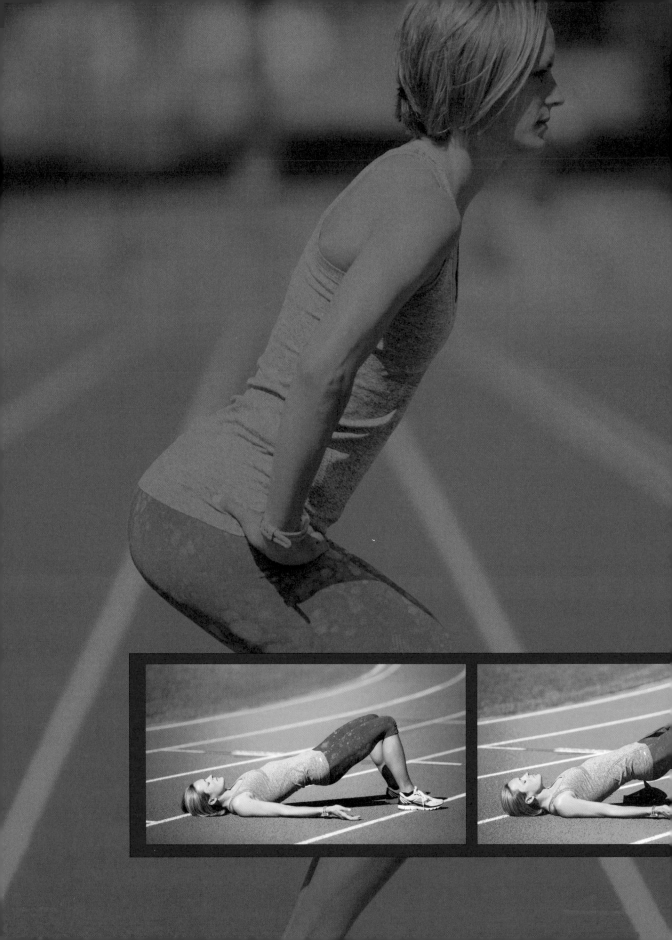

WAKE UP *YOUR* BUTT

The fact is, glute max is the boss of your push-off—the action of moving your body forward—in all physical pursuits. The biggest and strongest of your glutes, this guy adds power to your stride, pedal stroke, and more. However, because we're mostly forward-oriented, the quads (along with some other way-less-than-ideal helpers) tend to want to get in on the action more than they should. Countering the oh-so-common dominance of the quads—and the hamstrings' tendency to do more than they should—with specific focus on activating the glutes will optimize your power in any workout or sport.

Most of us impose an all-or-nothing approach with our glutes: We either go all out with buns of steel or totally hang out.

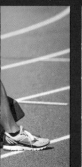
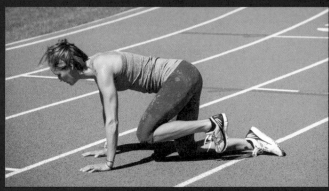
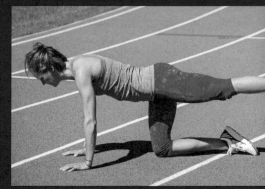

Glute clenching leads to strain

Don't walk around like a tight-ass. We can all squeeze our butt, but that doesn't mean we're skilled in engaging it properly. Here's a quick test: Get up, keep that booty clenched, and try to walk around and do some stuff. Does that clenching help or hinder your movement? You can't harness the power of your glutes to drive your forward motion when they're set in stone. Plus, when you clench your glutes you end up compressing your low back, which never ends well. Instead, you'll benefit way more from learning to isolate, activate, and fire your glutes to move better in sports and everyday life. Remember that clenching tight is just as bad as hanging out. By finding the middle ground—balanced, functional engagement—you optimize your effort.

✔ SOLUTION

WAKE-UP CALL

It's time to wake up your butt. Gluteus maximus (aka glute max) is what you need to activate and strengthen. Glute max is the largest of your glute muscles, so it makes sense that it should be doing the work. It occupies the bottom portion of each cheek. Focus on the place where your butt meets your hamstrings, and they will be easier to engage.

! PROBLEM

Lazy booty limits power

Despite their potential for power, the glutes are a commonly underused muscle group—they tend to be lazy. This problem sets off a chain reaction because when the glutes are not doing their job, muscles including the quads, hamstrings, the muscles around your low back, and even the calves have to work overtime, which can lead to all kinds of compensation pain and injuries.

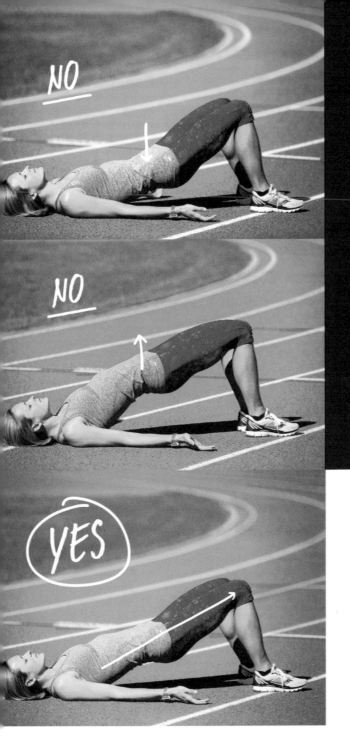

NO

NO

YES

ARE YOUR GLUTES WORKING TOO HARD OR NOT ENOUGH?

> Lie on your back with your knees bent, feet on the floor about hip width apart.

> Press down through your feet and lift your hips up so that your thighs and torso create a straight diagonal line from your knees to your shoulders.

> Bring one hand onto each butt cheek and cop a feel:

Are the muscles clenched hard, or are they soft?

Are they both engaged the same amount?

> Note your tendency.

✔ CORRECT

Instead of squeezing tight or just hanging out, try this:

> Engage glute max—the bottom part of each cheek, around where your butt meets your hamstrings. If that's elusive, use your hands to feel the muscles at work.

> Give it about 50 percent of your effort so that glute max doesn't clench but does its job.

> Feel for equal engagement between your right and left sides.

IT'S ALL ABOUT THE BOOTY

HIT RESET
TO WAKE UP YOUR BUTT

ROUTINE
✔ **Balance Your Booty** (p. 111)

BENEFITS

> Activate and strengthen your glutes so you can use them to full advantage

> Balance front/back body musculature of the lower body

> Add power to your stride

> Prevent low back pain

PRACTICE	Pre-workout/crosstraining
HOW LONG	Hold for 5-8 breaths or 10+ reps
PROPS	Block and strap, tie, or belt
RED FLAGS	Glute clenching Low back pain Spinal compensation

STRONG BUTT = STRONG STRIDE

TECHNIQUE
Use props to gather feedback

It can be hard to tell which muscles are working, especially when it comes to your less-used muscles. To gather more feedback, try breaking down Bridge (p. 111) and Chair (p. 114) with a block and a strap:

> Squeeze a yoga block widthwise between your shins, just above the knobby bones along the inside of your ankles.

> Loop a yoga strap (a tie or belt works, too) around the largest part of your thighs—it should be tight so that you can push your thighs into it.

> Notice how this feels—the opposing actions against the block and strap activate your muscles to effectively align your legs in neutral, optimizing their power.

Now repeat the poses sans props and see if you can engage your muscles the same way, even though you don't have the resistance to work against.

✔ BALANCE YOUR BOOTY

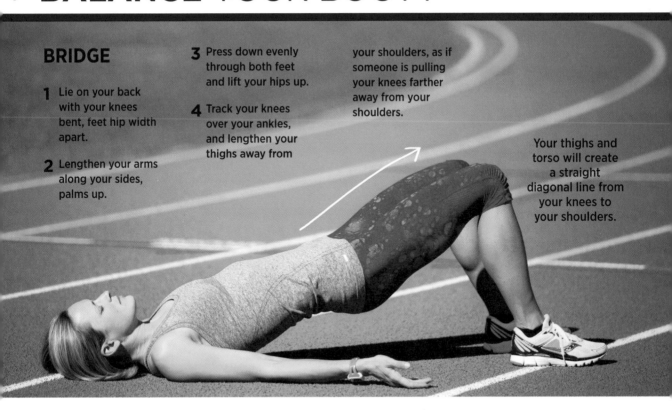

BRIDGE

1 Lie on your back with your knees bent, feet hip width apart.

2 Lengthen your arms along your sides, palms up.

3 Press down evenly through both feet and lift your hips up.

4 Track your knees over your ankles, and lengthen your thighs away from your shoulders, as if someone is pulling your knees farther away from your shoulders.

Your thighs and torso will create a straight diagonal line from your knees to your shoulders.

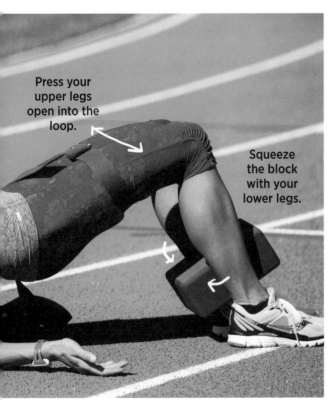

Press your upper legs open into the loop.

Squeeze the block with your lower legs.

FAQ But I thought I just had one butt?

Believe it or not, your butt is not one big muscle—you've got three glutes in each cheek. Glute max is the boss and should be powering your push-off, and glute med and glute min—the helpers—are there to help stabilize your hips so that you can get the most out of glute max. If you put your hands on your butt where your cheeks meet your legs and engage that lower portion, you're feeling the tone of glute max. Since this chapter is about powering your stride, glute max is our focus. The other guys, glute med and glute min, are covered in Mobilize & Stabilize Your Hips (p. 119).

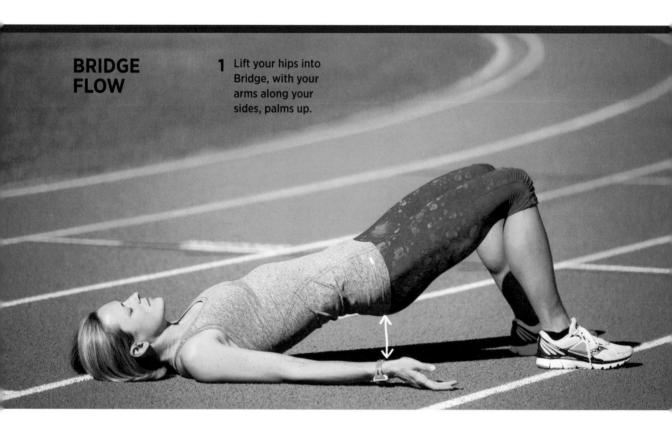

BRIDGE FLOW

1 Lift your hips into Bridge, with your arms along your sides, palms up.

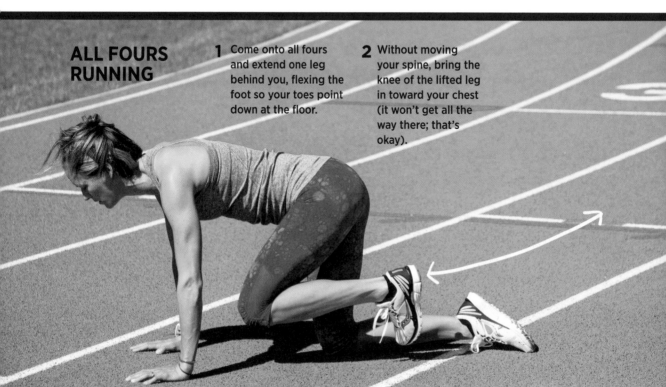

ALL FOURS RUNNING

1 Come onto all fours and extend one leg behind you, flexing the foot so your toes point down at the floor.

2 Without moving your spine, bring the knee of the lifted leg in toward your chest (it won't get all the way there; that's okay).

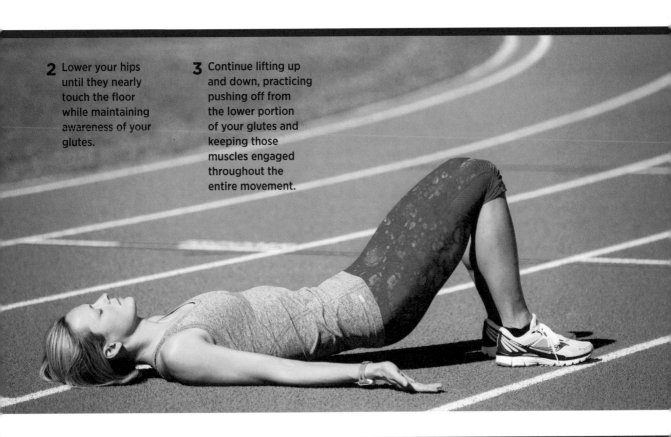

2 Lower your hips until they nearly touch the floor while maintaining awareness of your glutes.

3 Continue lifting up and down, practicing pushing off from the lower portion of your glutes and keeping those muscles engaged throughout the entire movement.

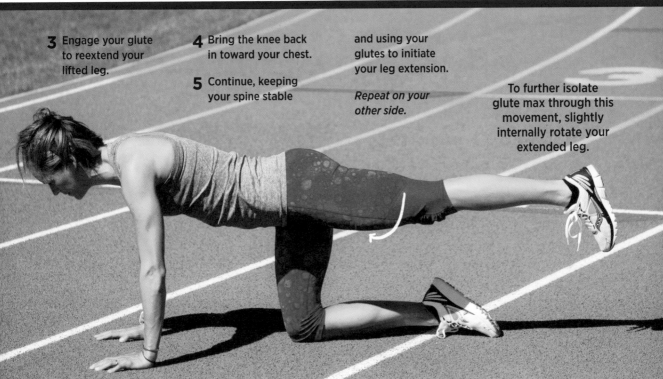

3 Engage your glute to reextend your lifted leg.

4 Bring the knee back in toward your chest.

5 Continue, keeping your spine stable and using your glutes to initiate your leg extension.

Repeat on your other side.

To further isolate glute max through this movement, slightly internally rotate your extended leg.

CHAIR

1 Establish a balanced foundation (p. 61) and bring your hands to your hips.

2 Bend your knees to come into a squat with your knees tracking in line with your ankles.

3 Focus on engaging your quads, hamstrings, and glutes evenly rather than relaxing your glutes and sticking your butt out behind you.

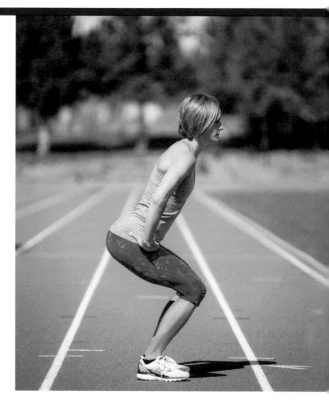

>> Remember to use props (p. 110) if you need more feedback about what's working.

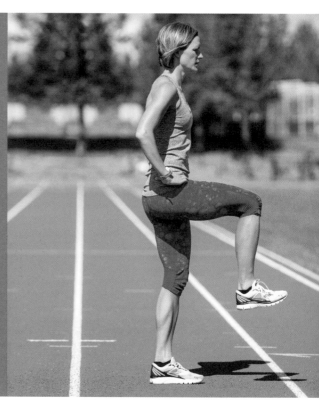

TECHNIQUE

Don't let your quads take over

When you're standing, and especially when you're balancing on one leg, you might feel more muscular engagement on the front of your thighs. It's super important to balance quad strength with equally strong, active glutes, so make sure your butt is working as much as your quads are—feel for the balance between front and back. If that's elusive, try putting more weight back into your heels as you shift your focus to the back of your body to encourage your glutes to fire—keep that awareness as you redistribute your weight evenly between front and back.

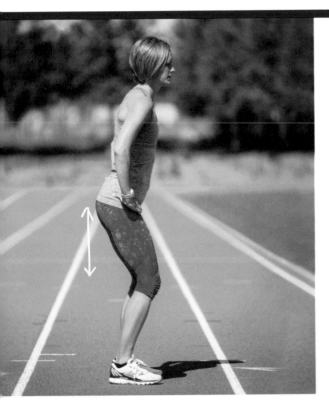

CHAIR FLOW

1 Set up Chair, pausing long enough to feel the muscles engage.

2 Rise to stand.

3 Bend your knees and return to Chair.

4 Move fluidly between Chair and standing—evenly engage the musculature of your legs and push off strongly with your glutes.

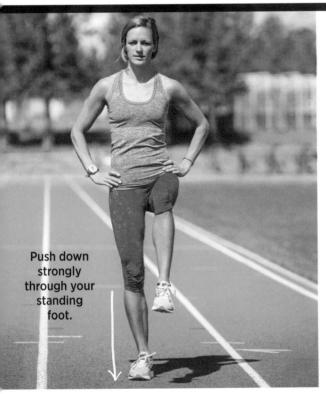

Push down strongly through your standing foot.

SINGLE-LEG BALANCE

1 Establish a balanced foundation and bring your hands to your hips.

2 Engage your core and lift one knee up to waist height, bending your knee to a 90-degree angle.

3 Hold here as you find your balance on your standing leg, keeping that standing knee slightly bent.

4 Feel the glute on your standing leg firing, as if you are about to push off.

Repeat on your other side.

GAME
PLAN

! My booty imbalance is:

✔ I'll wake up my glutes pre-workout by:

#hit**reset**
✔ What are you doing to wake up your butt today?

USE YOUR GLUTES

DO THE
**LITTLE
THINGS**

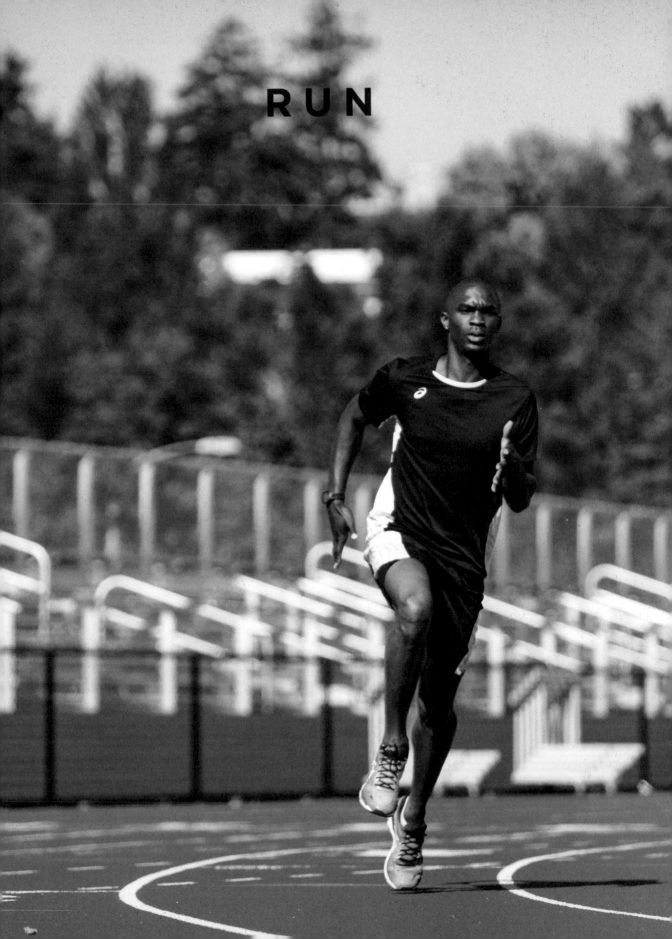

RUN

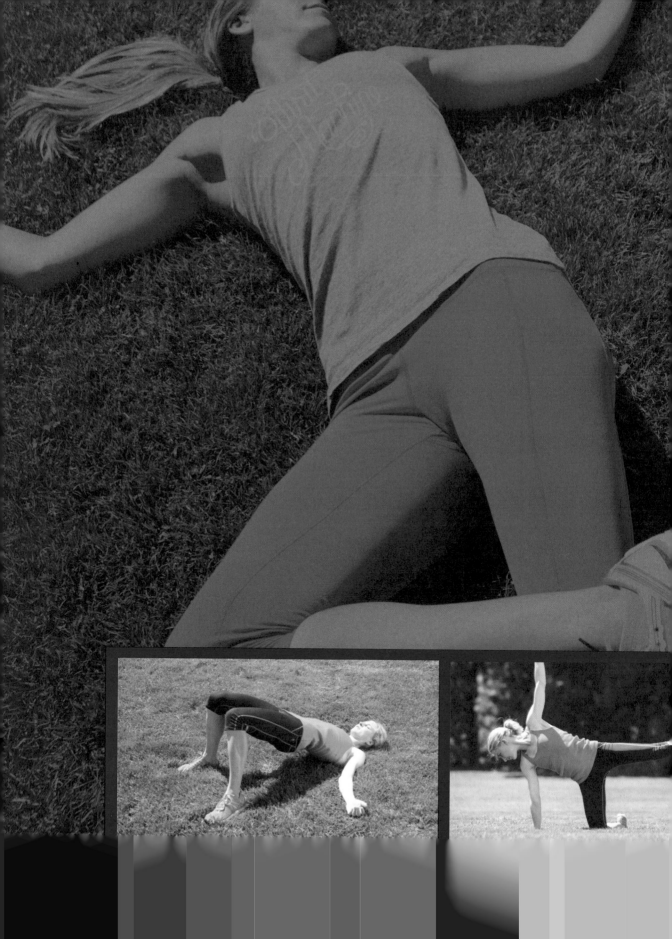

MOBILIZE & STABILIZE *YOUR* HIPS

Athletes often talk about needing to open up their hips. But what does that even mean? Here's the thing: Your hips are capable of a dynamic range of motion, but your typical forward-oriented movement neglects most of it. When you walk, run, or cycle, you only flex and extend your hips. Meanwhile, movement like rotation (turning out and in) and abduction and adduction (moving out to the side and back in) are rarely used, and as a result the hip muscles responsible for driving those movements become sleepy and tight. Ultimately, it's a balance of hip flexibility and strength—mobility and stability—that will help you prevent an array of injuries.

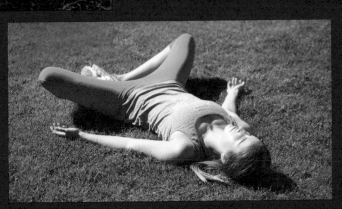

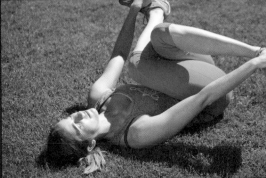

BE CLEAR ABOUT WHERE YOUR HIPS NEED OPENING

! PROBLEM

Limited hip mobility leads to strain in other areas

Your body will compensate for hip stiffness in all kinds of less-than-ideal ways. Aside from the general feeling of "booty lock," aka super-tight hip and glute muscles that impede your range of motion, lack of mobility is a common culprit behind everything from iliotibial band (IT band) pain—which usually leads to knee issues—to low back pain.

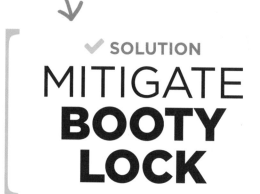

✔ **SOLUTION**

MITIGATE BOOTY LOCK

When it comes to hip mobility, it's use it or lose it. Optimal range of motion requires regular maintenance. Since most movement is forward-oriented (think walking, running, cycling ... even sitting!), you'll benefit immensely from giving extra attention to your non-habitual movement patterns such as rotation and moving side to side. And once you get some relief and enjoy more mobile hips, you'll be motivated to continue doing the consistent work that mitigates booty lock.

Weak hips are unstable

Obviously, the big muscles in your legs that propel you forward should be the most active. The problem is that the smaller, intrinsic muscles of your hips commonly forget how to do their job, which is to provide a foundation for optimal alignment so that the bigger muscles can do their job safely and effectively. What muscles are we talking about here? Glute med, glute min, and "the deep six"—a group of six little muscles that live deep in your hip, set up like spokes on a bicycle hub, wrapping around the top of your thighbone. When those muscles are doing their job effectively, they ultimately add power to your stride because the thighbones are stabilized in neutral in your hip joints.

A word of caution: Overstretching your hips can also lead to weakness, so be sure you devote equal time and attention to hip strength and flexibility. If you don't maintain your hip strength, it will be tough to keep moving forward as powerfully as possible. Especially when you're gassed, weakness in the hips can cause that area to flop from side to side, making you more likely to experience knee, hip, and back pain.

✔ SOLUTION

STRENGTHEN YOUR
HIP HELPERS

Changing up your usual forward motion with some lateral (side-to-side) action will help keep your hip stabilizers awake and strong so they can do their job of keeping your thighbones anchored in neutral.

WHERE DO YOUR **HIPS NEED OPENING?**

You should be able to internally (turn in) and externally (turn out) rotate your femur—your thighbone—about the same amount in each direction. Ideally, you'd also have the same range in both your right and your left hip. Use this self-test to help gauge which hip stretches will be the most beneficial for you.

> Sit with your knees bent, feet on the floor in front of you. Put your hands on the floor behind you for support.

> Pick up one leg, keeping the knee bent at about a 90-degree angle.

> Keeping your foot flexed, take your shin out away from the center of your body as far as you can—internally rotating your thigh in your hip joint—and notice where your range of motion stops.

> Still flexing your foot, take the same shin toward the center of your body as far as you can—externally rotating your thigh—and notice where your range of motion stops.

> Do this a couple times until it's pretty obvious which direction is tougher.

> Repeat on the other leg.

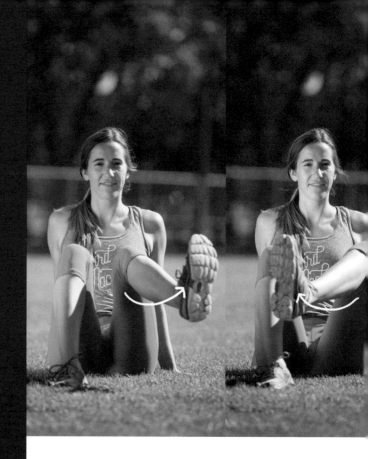

✔ CORRECT

After observing your internal and external rotation, you can generally assume that:

> If you're external-rotation dominant: You should spend more time on poses that encourage internal rotation, such as Reclined Hero (p. 125) and Flank (p. 126).

> If you're internal-rotation dominant: You should spend more time on poses that externally rotate, such as Figure 4 (p. 128) and Reclined Shoelace (p. 129).

> In general: Give a little extra love to whichever hip feels tighter—spend a few extra breaths on that side, or repeat some of the poses twice. Regardless of where you feel more limited, Reclined Windshield Wipers (p. 124) can help even out some of those imbalances and maintain fluidity in both hips.

HIT RESET TO MOBILIZE & STABILIZE YOUR HIPS

ROUTINES

- ✓ **Mitigate Booty Lock** (p. 123)
- ✓ **Strengthen Your Hip Helpers**
  (p. 132)

BENEFITS

> Maintain optimal range of motion in the hips

> Prevent back and IT band strain and compensation injuries

> Improve hip stability

> Ease muscular imbalances in the hips

PRACTICE	Pre-workout (Strengthen Your Hip Helpers) Post-workout/recovery (Mitigate Booty Lock)
HOW LONG	Hold for 5–8 breaths or 10+ reps/multiple sets for movement
PROPS	Blocks or pillows
RED FLAGS	Knee injuries Spinal compensation

✓ MITIGATE **BOOTY LOCK**

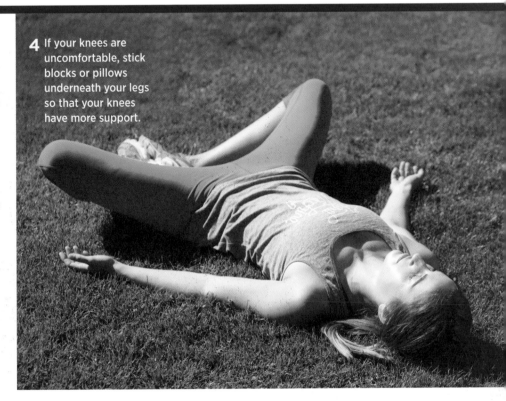

RECLINED BUTTERFLY

1 Lie on your back and extend your arms along your sides, palms up.

2 Bring the soles of your feet together and drop your thighs toward the floor.

3 Feel the stretch along the inseam of your upper legs and into your hips— if it's too intense, move your feet farther away from your body.

4 If your knees are uncomfortable, stick blocks or pillows underneath your legs so that your knees have more support.

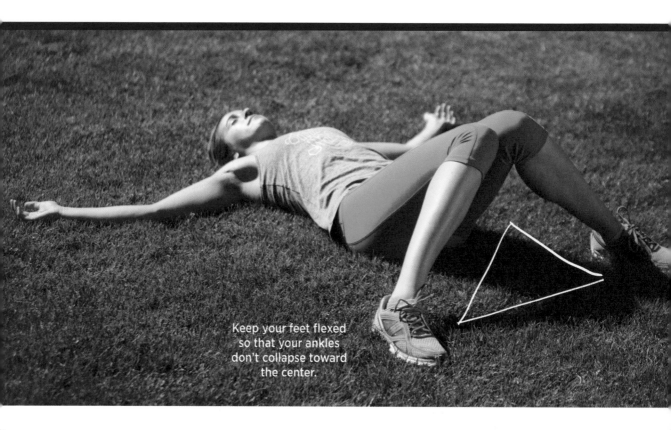

Keep your feet flexed so that your ankles don't collapse toward the center.

RECLINED WINDSHIELD WIPERS

1 From Reclined Hero, separate your knees.

2 Drop your knees to one side and turn your head to look to the opposite side.

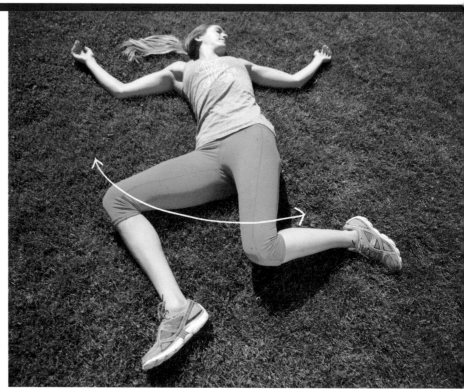

RECLINED HERO

1 Lie on your back and extend your arms open to the sides about shoulder height, palms up.

2 Bring your feet wider than hip width (about as wide as your mat if you're using one) and drop your thighs together into a triangle shape.

3 See if you can take your feet another inch away from each other, so the knees might not even be touching, and feel the space that's created in your hip joints and around your low back.

UNLOCK YOUR HIPS

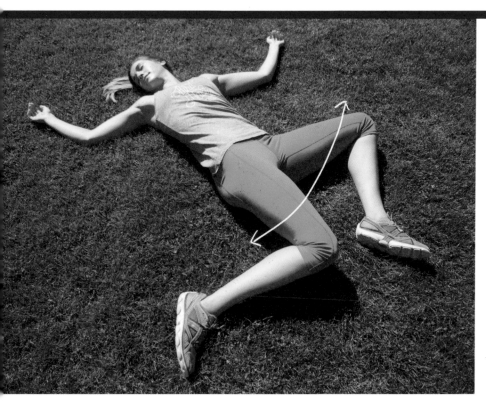

3 Lift your knees back to center, then drop them to the other side and look in the opposite direction.

4 Continue, just like windshield wipers moving side to side.

Do this sequence of poses first on one side, then pause and feel the difference before repeating the sequence on your other side.

FLANK

1 Lie on your back and extend your arms open to the sides at shoulder height, palms up.

2 Bring your feet wider than hip width apart and drop your thighs to one side.

3 Put your foot on top of the other thigh, using the weight of that leg to encourage the thigh to rotate farther in the hip joint and drop toward the floor.

4 If it feels too hard to keep your foot on the other leg or if either of your knees are uncomfortable, just rest your foot on the floor instead.

5 Keep both feet flexed.

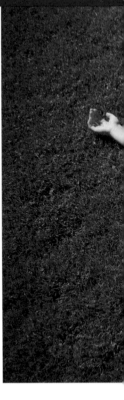

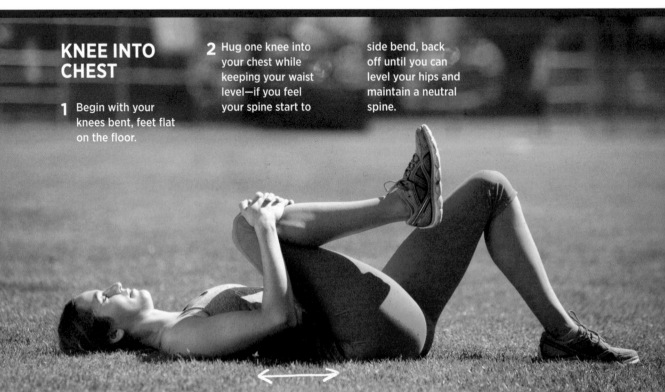

KNEE INTO CHEST

1 Begin with your knees bent, feet flat on the floor.

2 Hug one knee into your chest while keeping your waist level—if you feel your spine start to side bend, back off until you can level your hips and maintain a neutral spine.

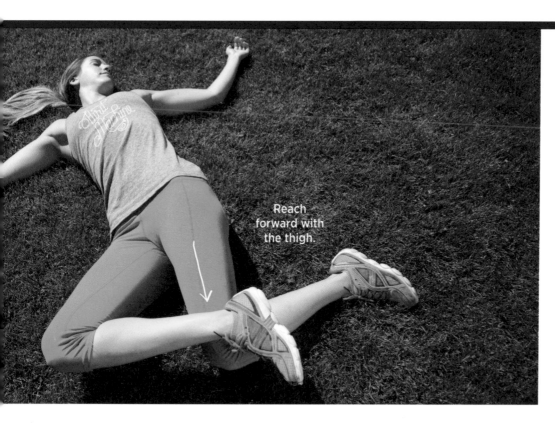

Reach forward with the thigh.

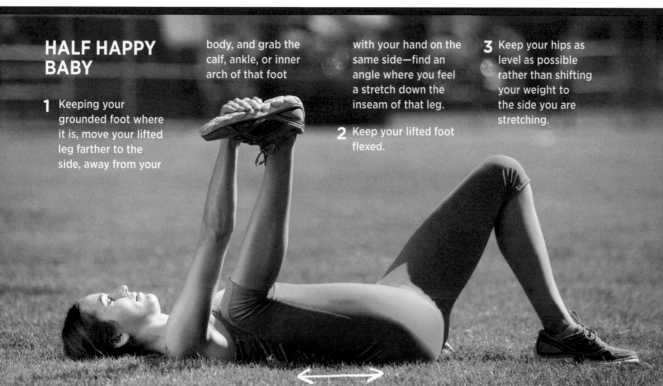

HALF HAPPY BABY

1 Keeping your grounded foot where it is, move your lifted leg farther to the side, away from your body, and grab the calf, ankle, or inner arch of that foot with your hand on the same side—find an angle where you feel a stretch down the inseam of that leg.

2 Keep your lifted foot flexed.

3 Keep your hips as level as possible rather than shifting your weight to the side you are stretching.

FIGURE 4

1 From Half Happy Baby, cross your ankle over the opposite knee, keeping the foot flexed.

2 Stay here or pick your legs up, interlacing your fingers around your bottom leg hamstrings or shin.

3 Make sure both sides of your waist are even—if you feel your spine start to side bend, slide the foot that's on the floor farther away from your body until you can level your hips and maintain a neutral spine.

4 Add a little rock side to side. It's small. Notice how the stretch changes as you change the angles. Use that small movement to encourage more fluidity around the hip joint.

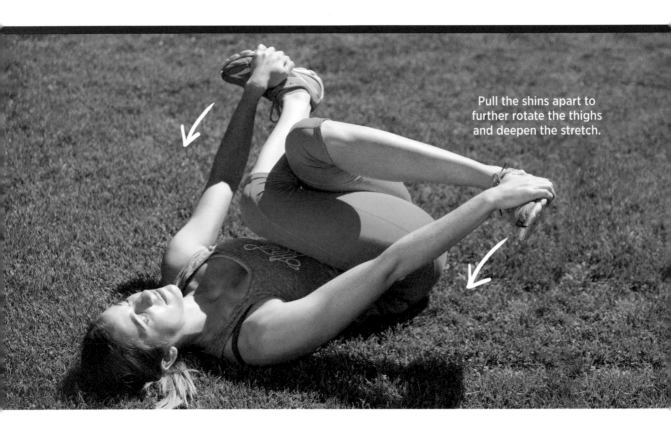

Pull the shins apart to further rotate the thighs and deepen the stretch.

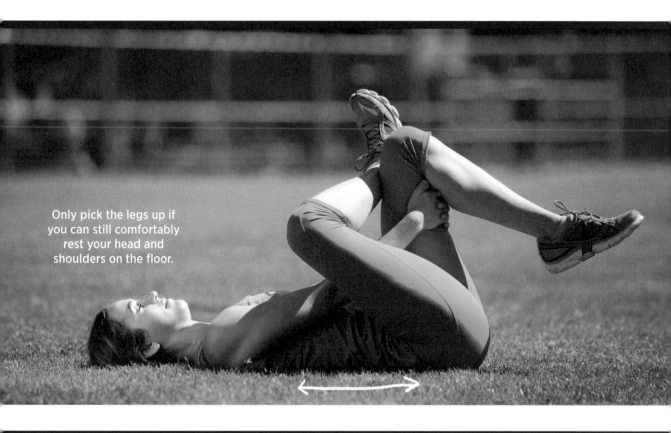

Only pick the legs up if you can still comfortably rest your head and shoulders on the floor.

RECLINED SHOELACE

1 From Figure 4, cross one knee over your other knee.

2 Hug those crossed legs into your chest, holding whatever you can reach and keeping your butt as level as possible against the floor.

3 Keep both feet flexed. If you feel it in your knees, back off, or if it's a struggle in general, return to Figure 4.

STRETCH THE WAY YOU WANT TO FEEL— FLUID, NOT RIGID

 Pause and feel the difference between sides before returning to Flank and doing the sequence on your other side.

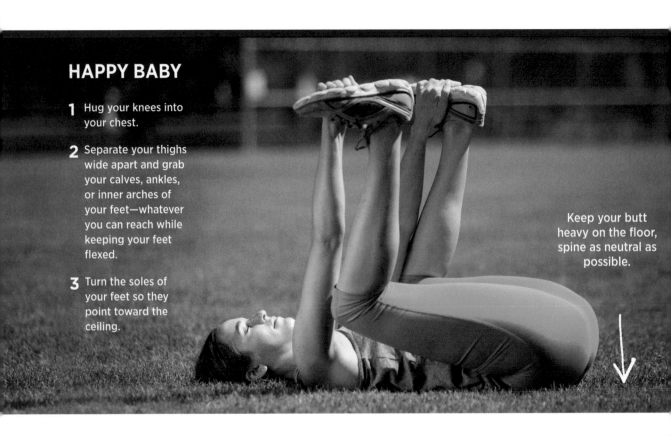

HAPPY BABY

1 Hug your knees into your chest.

2 Separate your thighs wide apart and grab your calves, ankles, or inner arches of your feet—whatever you can reach while keeping your feet flexed.

3 Turn the soles of your feet so they point toward the ceiling.

Keep your butt heavy on the floor, spine as neutral as possible.

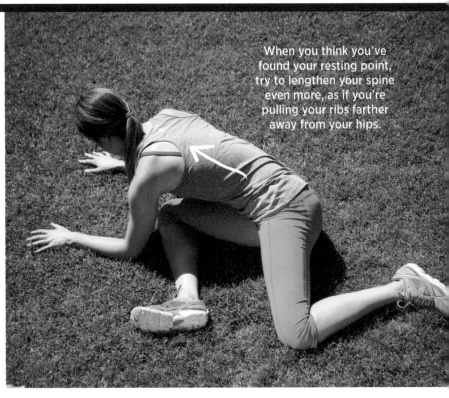

BONUS

PINWHEEL

1 Sit down and bend your knees, staggering one leg in front of the other so that they make a pinwheel shape, with a little bit of space between your front foot and your back knee.

2 Keep both feet flexed.

3 Sit up tall and turn your torso toward your front thigh, and lie down on top of it, propping yourself up on your forearms.

Repeat on your other side.

When you think you've found your resting point, try to lengthen your spine even more, as if you're pulling your ribs farther away from your hips.

FAQ Will stretching make me lose my hops?

This is an old-school mind-set that leaves all you fast-twitchers—sprinters, jumpers, ballers, and lovers of any activity requiring explosive movement—uptight. Long story short, we all have fast- and slow-twitch muscles, which are influenced by genetics and the type of training we're doing. Especially when it comes to passive stretching (the bulk of the Resets in this routine), we tend to focus on slower-twitch and stability muscles, which have a significant impact on how much of your true muscular power you can tap. Regardless of your muscle makeup, if slow-twitch muscles are tight and dry and your glutes are locked, the circulation to fast-twitch muscles will decrease.

The fact is that tight connective tissue doesn't equate to elastic bounce—it simply reduces blood flow and nerve function, which definitely isn't going to help your vertical. When connective tissue is tight and circulation to your calves is compromised, your nerves will not be able to communicate as well with those muscles. In other words, when your fast-twitch muscles aren't getting proper circulation, you lose some of your explosive potential. Improve your fluidity and your circulation with regular stretching, and the nerves will start talking to your muscles loud and clear, giving you every advantage when it comes to your ups. Think about it: Are you skipping a massage because you're scared it will ruin your bounce?

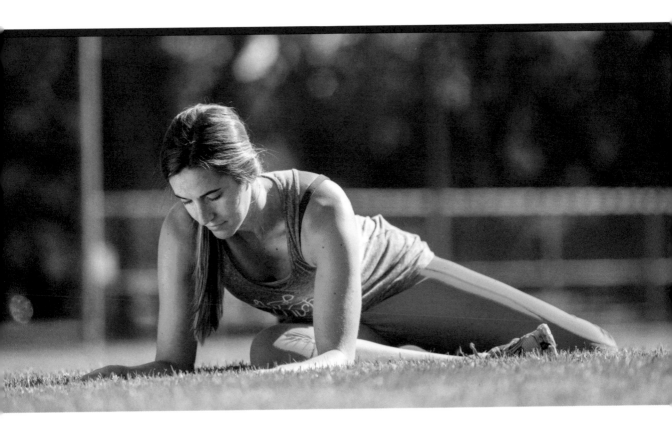

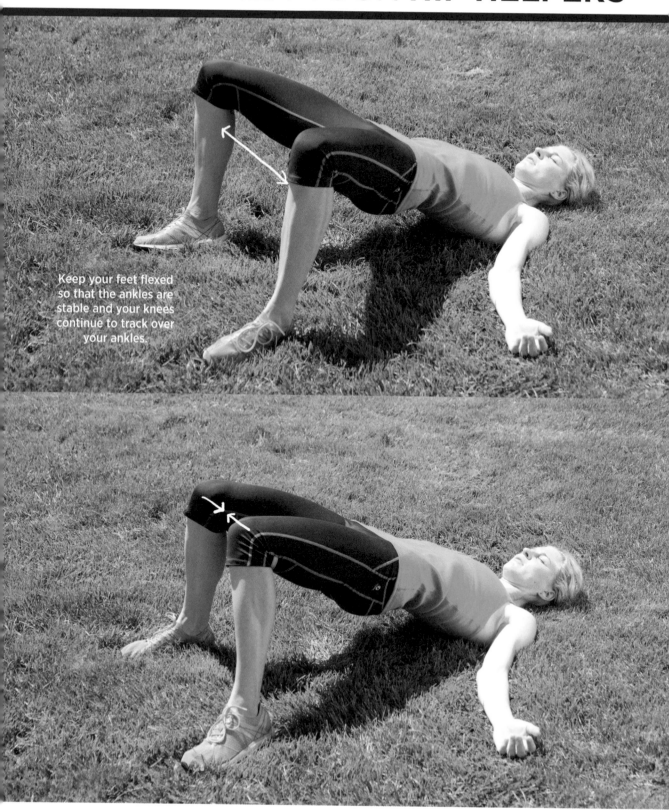

Keep your feet flexed so that the ankles are stable and your knees continue to track over your ankles.

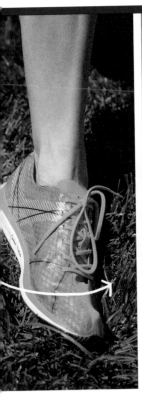
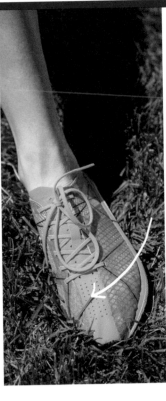

WIDE BRIDGE FLOW

1 Lie down with your knees bent and bring your feet wider than hip width apart and parallel. Extend your arms along your sides, palms up.

2 Press down through your feet and lift your hips into Bridge (p. 111).

3 Keeping your hips lifted, rock toward the outer edges of your feet so that your knees move apart.

4 Bring your knees toward each other as you rock inward to the arches of your feet.

5 Continue ...

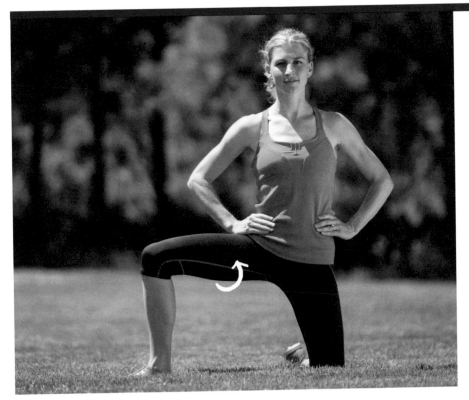

WARRIOR 2 PREP

1 Kneel and extend one leg out to the side, knee bent like a kickstand—put some padding under your supporting knee if necessary.

2 Rotate your thigh on the extended leg so that your foot points perpendicular to your body, and keep the knee tracking over the ankle.

3 Put your hands on your hips.

Repeat on your other side.

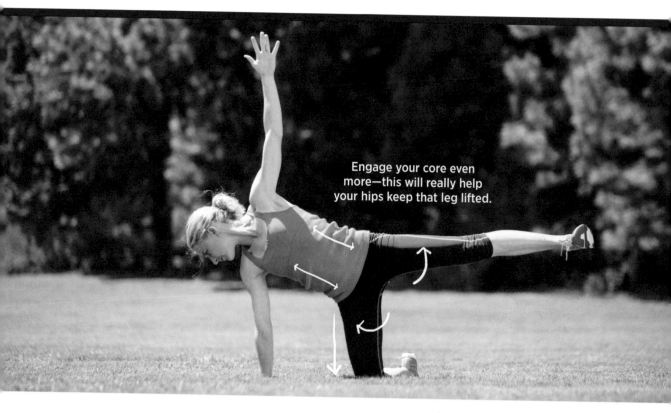

Engage your core even more—this will really help your hips keep that leg lifted.

HALF MOON PREP

1 Kneel and extend one leg out to the side like a kickstand, keeping your toes pointing forward and foot flat—put some padding under your supporting knee if needed.

2 Bring your torso into alignment with your kneeling leg and rest the hand on the kneeling side on the floor or a block— make sure you're not straining to reach the floor.

3 Extend your other arm up and reach through your fingers so that the arm feels active, as if someone is pulling it toward the ceiling.

4 Your supporting hand and knee should pretty much make a straight line with your foot on the extended leg.

5 Engage your core and see if you can lengthen your spine more, creating more space between your ribs and hips.

6 Lift your leg up, bringing it parallel to the floor, and feel the work happening deep in your hips.

Repeat on your other side.

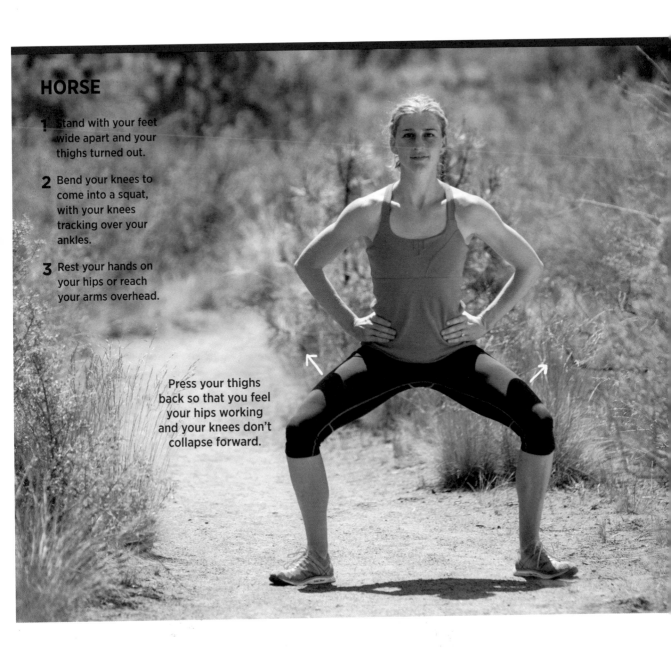

HORSE

1 Stand with your feet wide apart and your thighs turned out.

2 Bend your knees to come into a squat, with your knees tracking over your ankles.

3 Rest your hands on your hips or reach your arms overhead.

Press your thighs back so that you feel your hips working and your knees don't collapse forward.

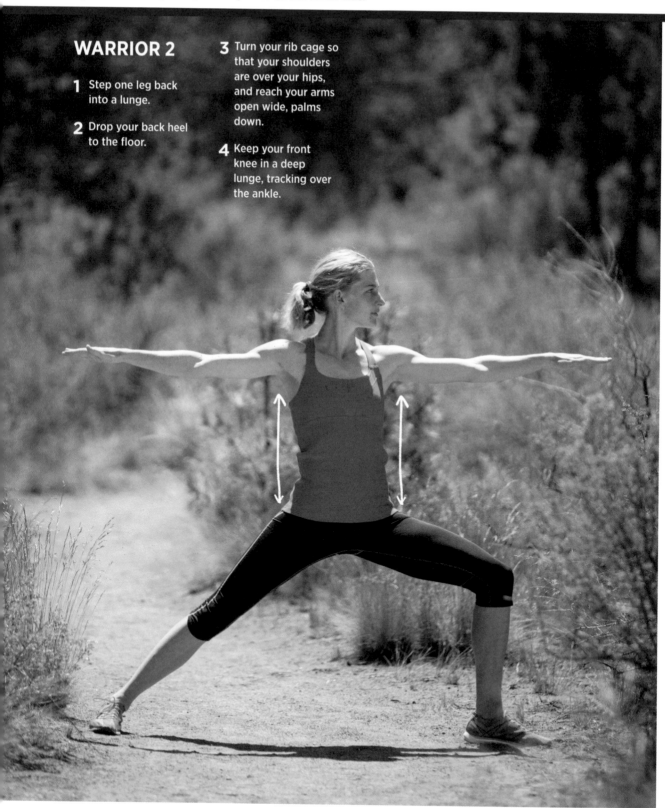

WARRIOR 2

1 Step one leg back into a lunge.

2 Drop your back heel to the floor.

3 Turn your rib cage so that your shoulders are over your hips, and reach your arms open wide, palms down.

4 Keep your front knee in a deep lunge, tracking over the ankle.

TREE PREP

1 Establish a balanced foundation (p. 61) wand bring your hands to your hips.

2 Engage your core and lift your knee up to hip height, bending your knee at a 90-degree angle.

3 Keeping your hips and spine where they are, move your lifted leg out to the side, away from your body (keeping it near hip height), and stopping when you feel the natural end of your range of motion.

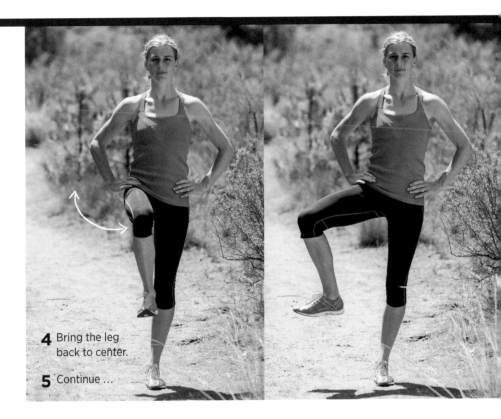

4 Bring the leg back to center.

5 Continue ...

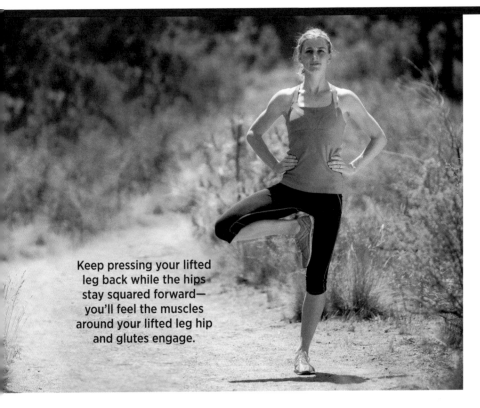

Keep pressing your lifted leg back while the hips stay squared forward—you'll feel the muscles around your lifted leg hip and glutes engage.

TREE

1 From Tree Prep, slide the sole of your foot up your leg, resting it on your ankle or calf (feel free to keep the ball of your foot on the floor for added stability).

2 Bring the sole of the foot up onto the inner thigh. Make sure to keep your foot off the knee of your standing leg.

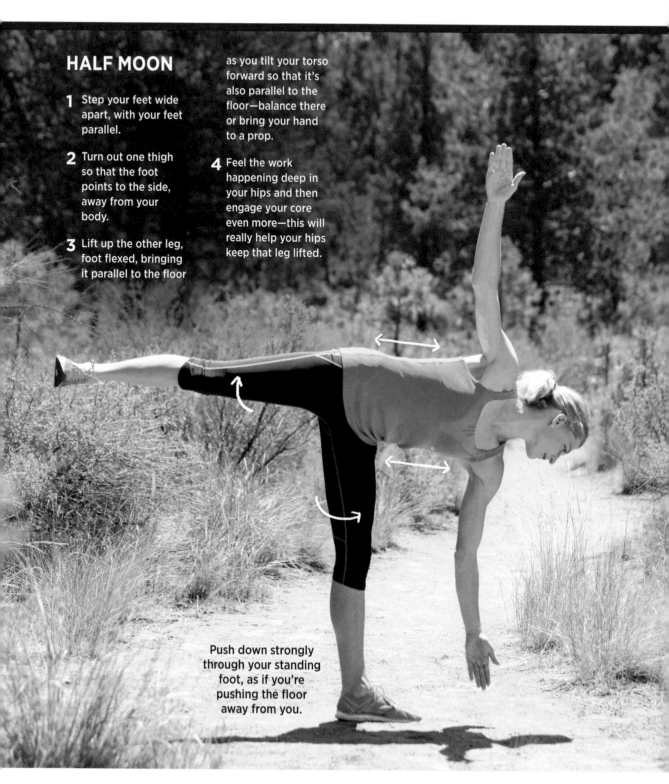

HALF MOON

1 Step your feet wide apart, with your feet parallel.

2 Turn out one thigh so that the foot points to the side, away from your body.

3 Lift up the other leg, foot flexed, bringing it parallel to the floor

as you tilt your torso forward so that it's also parallel to the floor—balance there or bring your hand to a prop.

4 Feel the work happening deep in your hips and then engage your core even more—this will really help your hips keep that leg lifted.

Push down strongly through your standing foot, as if you're pushing the floor away from you.

Pause and feel the difference between sides before returning to Warrior 2 and doing the sequence on your other side.

GAME
PLAN

! Where my hips need opening:

! Where my hips need strengthening:

✓ I'll balance my hip mobility and stability by:

#hitreset

✓ What are you doing to mobilize and stabilize your hips today?

MOVE SIDE TO SIDE

DO THE
**LITTLE
THINGS**

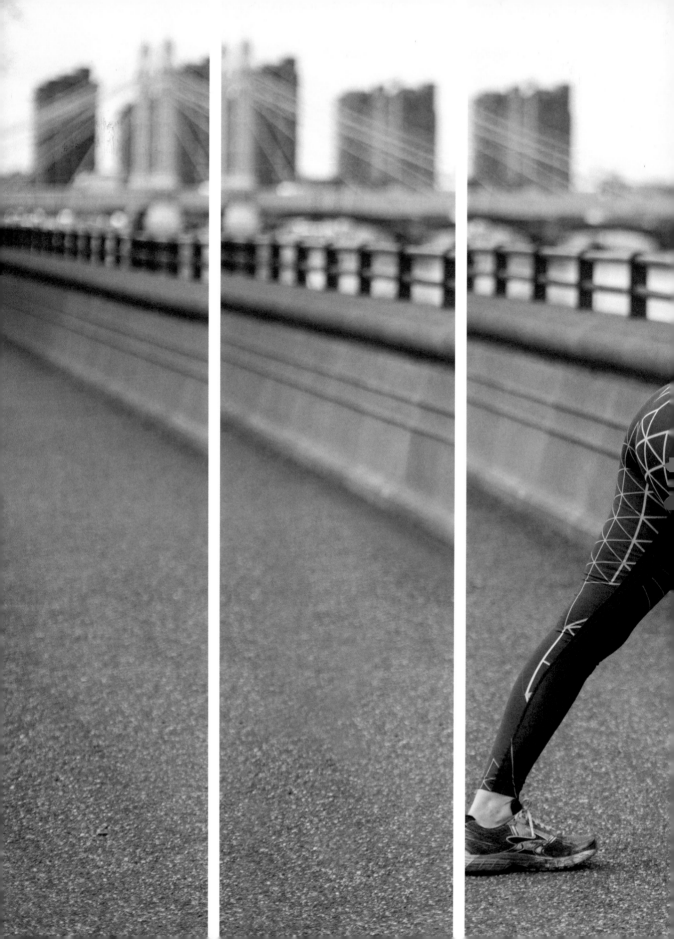

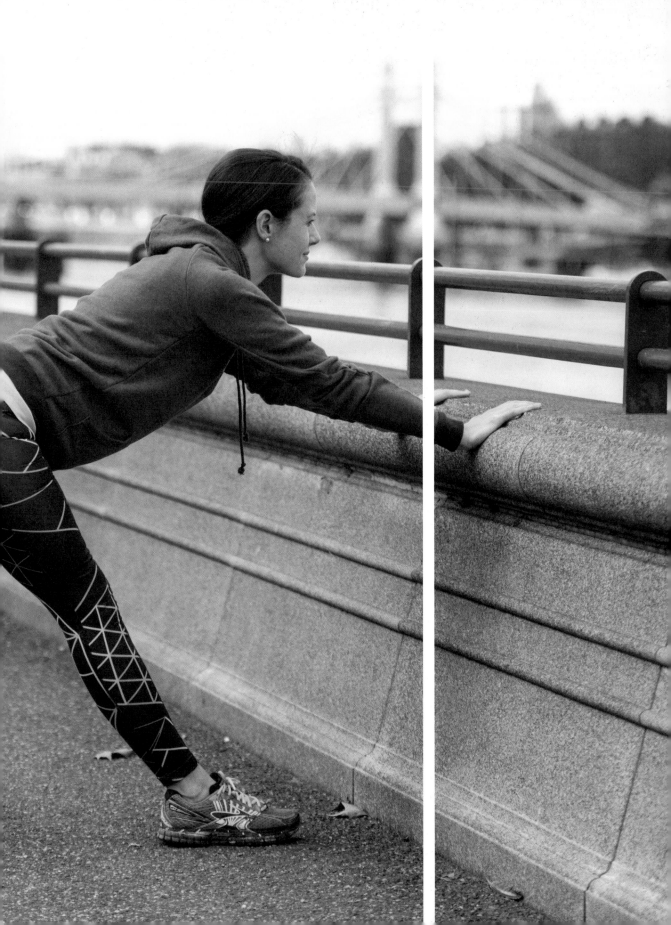

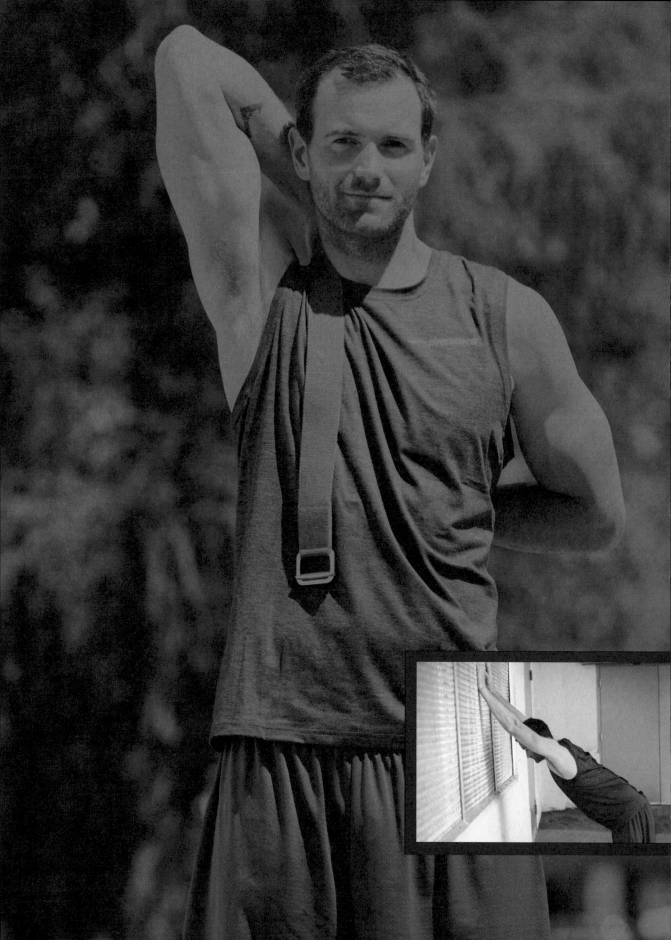

SORT OUT *YOUR* SHOULDERS

There's a lot going on in your shoulders. Despite what you might think, each of your shoulders is made of two joints:

> The ball and socket, where your upper arm meets your shoulder blade—the glenohumeral (GH) joint

> The shoulder blade, where it sits on the back of your rib cage—the scapulothoracic (ST) joint

In other words, your shoulder isn't just one big junction where your arm meets your body. Instead, these two key joints and the surrounding muscles work together to control the complex movement of your arms and shoulder blades. Awareness of proper alignment, as well as a balance of flexibility and strength, is what will help you maintain good posture and prevent a range of issues—from upper back soreness to rotator cuff injuries.

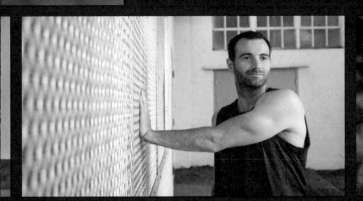
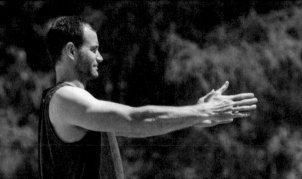

Stiff chest pulls you forward

Most athletic activities tighten your pectorals (the muscles of your chest) and reinforce the forward-flopping posture you've cultivated during all your sitting, plus compress the front of your GH joint (the ball and socket). No matter what you're doing, it's impossible to maintain optimal upper body posture and form with short, stiff pecs.

✔ SOLUTION

STRETCH YOUR CHEST

Clearly, we all need to relengthen the front of our torsos. But in order to effectively stretch rather than strain your oh-so-critical pecs, you've got to get your shoulder blades back into the right place. Guiding your scapula into their home on your upper back so that you can safely open the space across your chest will help you get your upper bod back into balance, not only reducing your injury risk but also optimizing your form and increasing your power when you run up a hill or stroke through open water.

REMIND YOUR SHOULDER BLADES WHERE THEIR HOME IS

FIND YOUR
BACK PACK

You know that stiff "I need to stretch my upper back" feeling? Despite the lack of ease you might feel in that area, it's more likely that your upper back is already overstretched. Don't be deceived by this sensation: The feeling of soreness from being overstretched can be very similar to the feeling of soreness from being overengaged, because both result from overuse.

While you might feel like you need a stretch back there, what will actually bring you relief and help to neutralize your structure is some work that first gets your shoulder blades back into optimal alignment and then strengthens your upper back muscles to keep them there. Couple the bonus pose on page 156 with the Find Your Back Pack routine (p. 50) to get the job done.

! PROBLEM

Overstretched upper back is weak & unstable

Depending on what you're trying to do with your arms, your shoulder blades—and ST joint—either need to move or be stable. For example, when you do push-ups, your shoulder blades need to be stable on your upper back, whereas when you swim freestyle, your shoulder blades must access a big range of motion. However, the forward-flopping posture that results from stiff pecs pulls the shoulder blades way outside their optimal alignment, creating weakness and instability that increase injury risk.

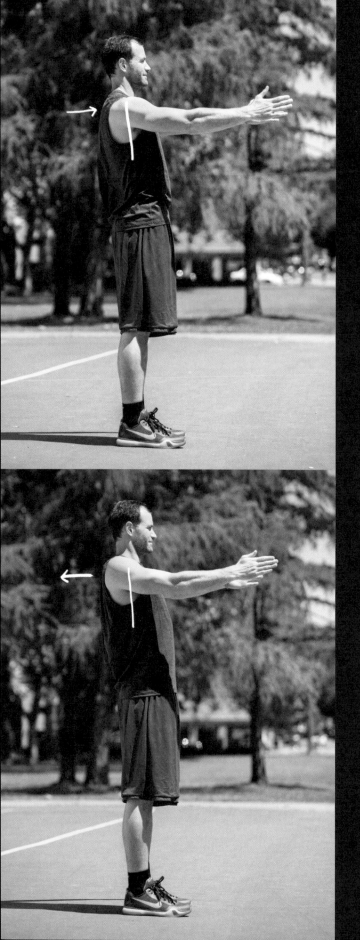

WHERE ARE YOUR
SHOULDER BLADES?

> Stand in profile in front of a mirror and extend your arms in front of you so that they're parallel to the floor with your palms facing each other.

> Keeping your head where it is (don't let it move forward), reach your arms forward so that your upper back broadens and your shoulder blades move apart.

> Squeeze your shoulder blades together, moving your arms back so that your chest broadens.

> Do a few more rounds, feeling the range of motion available to your shoulder blades.

> Come to stillness and notice where they naturally settle.

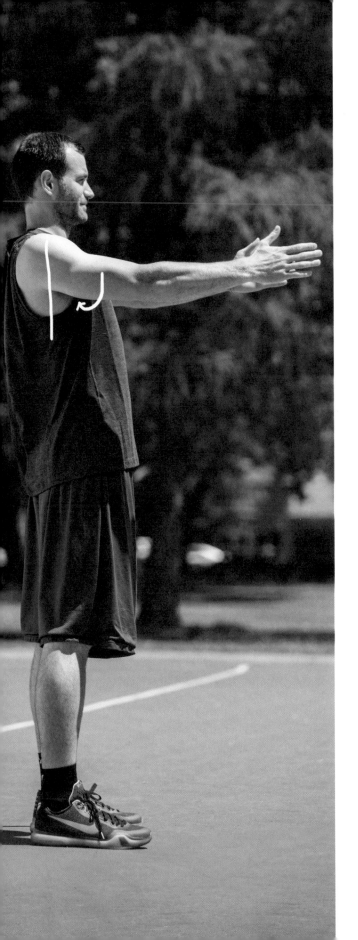

✔ CORRECT

Find neutral—where your shoulder blades are stable on your upper back so that your shoulders move back and your chest is spacious.

> ❯ Release your arms along your sides and externally rotate your upper arm bones (imagine you're turning a doorknob), and you'll feel your shoulder blades really anchor into place (p. 149).

> ❯ This is optimal and where things need to be so that you can safely and effectively coordinate the movement of your two shoulder joints.

Use this simple exercise (aka Shoulder Row) whenever you need a reminder about where neutral alignment is or when your shoulders and/or upper back feel tense.

HIT RESET TO SORT OUT YOUR SHOULDERS

ROUTINES

✔ **Stretch Your Chest** (p. 150)

✔ **Find Your Back Pack** (p. 50)
   + bonus pose (p. 156)

BENEFITS

❯ Maintain optimal range of motion in the shoulders

❯ Increase shoulder stability

❯ Improve posture

❯ Prevent shoulder strain and compensation injuries

❯ Ease muscular imbalances

PRACTICE	Post-workout/recovery
HOW LONG	Hold for 5–8 breaths or 10+ reps/multiple sets for movement
PROPS	Strap, tie, or belt
RED FLAGS	Shoulder injuries Spinal compensation via side bending, back bending, or rounding forward

MORE SPACE ACROSS YOUR CHEST = MORE ENERGY

Externally rotate your upper arm bones

Keep in mind that you've got to get your shoulder blades into the right place before you can access an optimal range of motion with your arms. One of the best ways to ensure this is to externally rotate your upper arm bones before doing anything else—especially before you reach your arms overhead. Here's how:

1 Stand with your arms along your sides.

2 Externally rotate your upper arm bones and turn your palms forward as if you were turning a doorknob—this will make your elbows point straight back (instead of out to the side).

3 Notice how when you do this, the muscles around your shoulder blades engage and move in and down toward the center of your upper back.

4 Notice also how this creates more space across your chest.

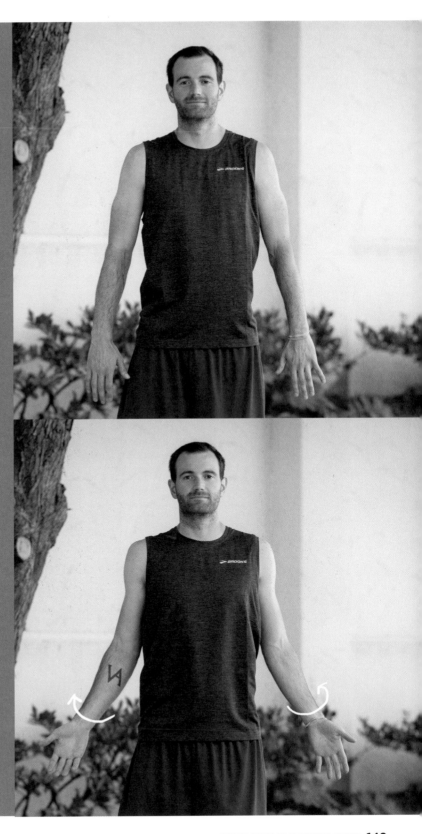

STRETCH YOUR **CHEST**

**SHOULDER
CIRCLES**

1 This is just what it sounds like—circle your shoulders!

2 Feel your shoulder blades glide freely around your upper back as you gradually create more space across your chest.

3 Do 5–10 circles in each direction, keeping your neck relaxed.

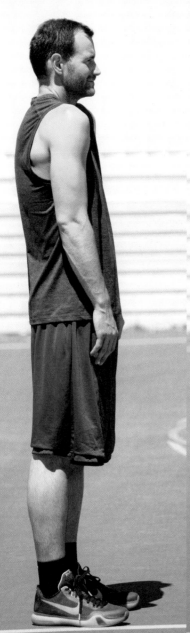

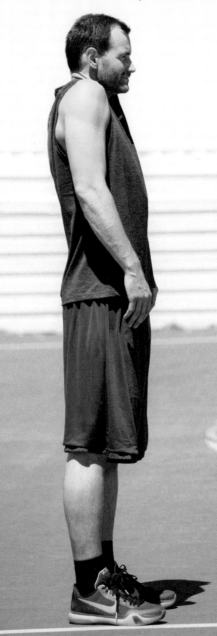

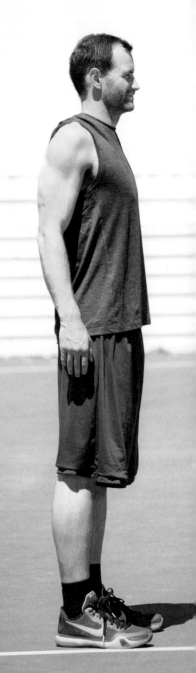

CHEST EXPANSION

1 Bring your hands to your low back and interlace your fingers—if that's not possible, rest your hands on your low back with your fingers pointing toward the floor.

2 Squeeze your shoulder blades toward each other and move your elbows closer together so you feel your chest broaden.

3 Use deeper breathing to deepen the stretch, as if you're trying to puff up your chest with your inhale.

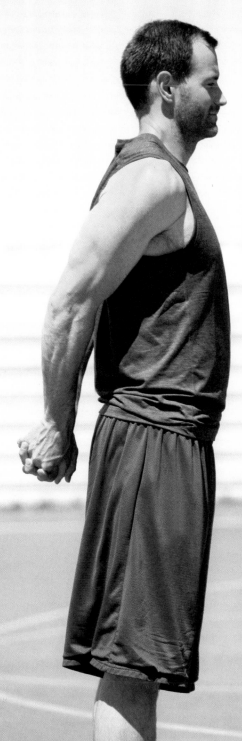

Feel the stretch across the front of your chest and the fronts of your shoulders as your shoulder blades continue to move together.

MOVING GOALPOST

1 Hold your strap with one end in each hand. If it's unwieldy, fold it in half.

2 Bring your strap overhead so you're making a big Y shape—if that feels hard, separate your hands farther.

3 Keeping your hands where they are, pull them away from each other so that you feel some tone in your shoulders and chest.

4 Bend your elbows and bring your strap behind your head.

5 Keep your core engaged and front ribs moving toward each other to help maintain a neutral spine and avoid back bending (your ribs popping open is a good sign that's happening).

6 Straighten your arms back to a Y.

7 Bend the elbows again and continue the movement.

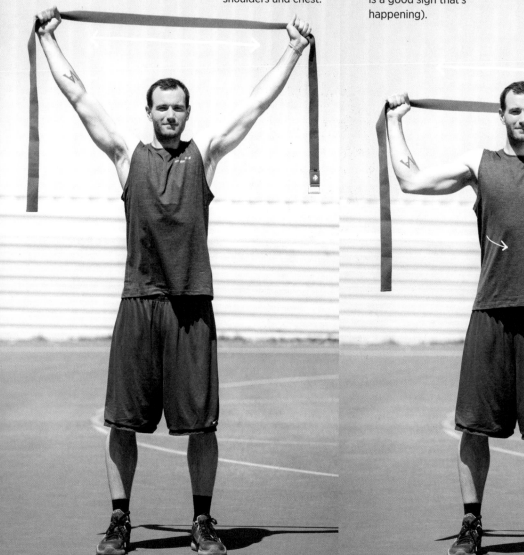

ROTATOR CUFF STRETCH

1 Hold your strap in one hand behind your head, elbow bent and pointing toward the ceiling, so that your strap dangles behind you.

2 Reach your other arm behind you to grab the strap.

3 Pull down on the strap to encourage the top arm to move farther, deepening the stretch you feel in the back of your upper arm.

4 Keep your core engaged to help avoid back bending.

Repeat on your other side.

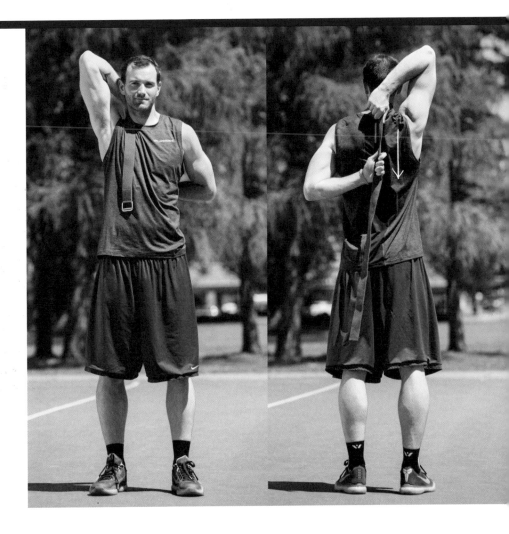

FAQ What's going on with my rotator cuff?

There seems to be some confusion about the famous rotator cuff. Despite what you might think, it's not one specific muscle. Rather, the "cuff" is a group of four muscles that hold the top of your upper arm bone against your shoulder blade. Your rotator cuff includes:

supraspinatus	infraspinatus
teres major	subscapularis

You've probably heard of the dreaded rotator cuff tear. This injury is actually more likely to be a tear in the labrum, which is a ring of cartilage that borders the shoulder socket. Regardless, this injury is common in many sports, which isn't surprising given the force you exert on this area when you swim butterfly or serve a tennis ball. It can be a major pain. One of the best ways to avoid rotator cuff issues is to learn to effectively coordinate the movement of your shoulder blades and arm bones. That's what we're practicing in this chapter.

WALL CHEST STRETCH

1 Stand perpendicular to a wall with a balanced foundation (p. 61).

2 With the arm closest to the wall, turn out your upper arm bone as if you've just turned a doorknob with your hand—you should feel your shoulder blade on that side move in and down toward the center of your upper back.

3 Keep that shoulder blade where it is and place your hand on the wall about a foot behind you at shoulder height—engage your core to maintain a neutral spine.

4 Press into the wall with your hand and straighten your arm without locking your elbow.

5 Rotate your rib cage away from the wall to deepen the stretch.

Repeat on your other side.

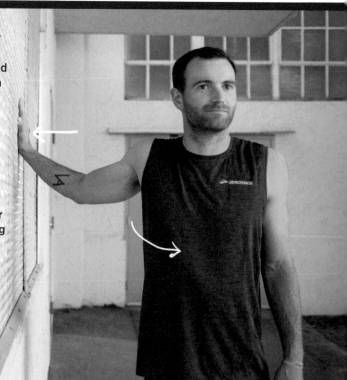

HALF DRAGONFLY AT THE WALL

1 Stand perpendicular to a wall with a balanced foundation, and reach across your body to put your palm flat on the wall at shoulder height with your fingers pointing up.

2 Bring your other shoulder (that's closest to the wall) as close to your working arm as possible.

3 Keep pressing your hand into the wall and relax your neck.

Repeat on your other side.

Draw the shoulder blade of your extended arm in and down toward the center of your upper back.

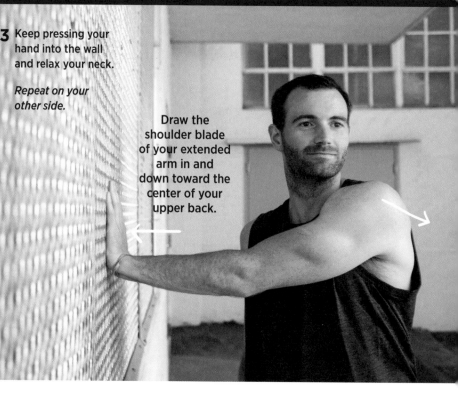

SHOWER

1 Face the wall and put your hands onto the wall about an arm's length above your shoulders, with your fingers pointing toward the ceiling.

2 Step your feet a few feet back from the wall and lengthen your spine toward the floor.

3 Engage your core and lift your ribs together to avoid collapsing your mid-spine toward the floor.

4 Look at the place where the wall and floor meet to help your neck find a comfortable neutral position.

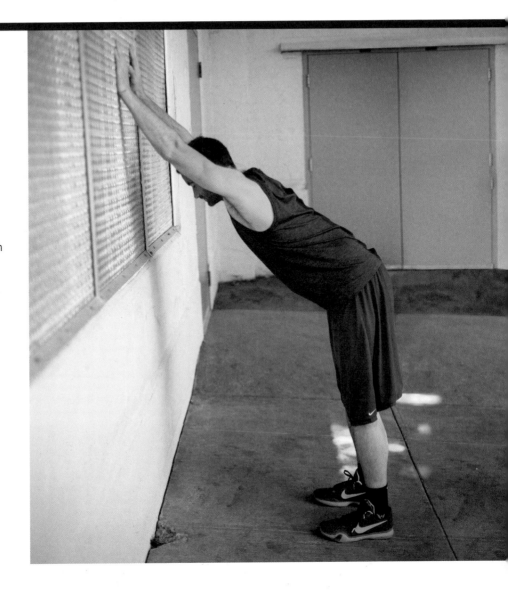

BONUS

SHOULDER T

1 Stand with a balanced foundation and externally rotate your upper arm bones so that your palms face forward.

2 Keep your shoulder blades where they are as you lift your arms to shoulder height with your palms facing up.

3 Continue to focus on the work happening in your upper back as those muscles gain strength to stabilize your shoulder blades into their home.

4 Keep your core engaged to maintain a neutral spine.

5 Hold for 2–5(+) minutes!

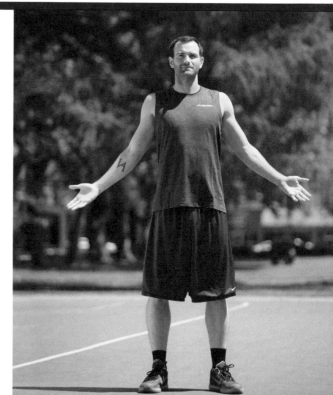

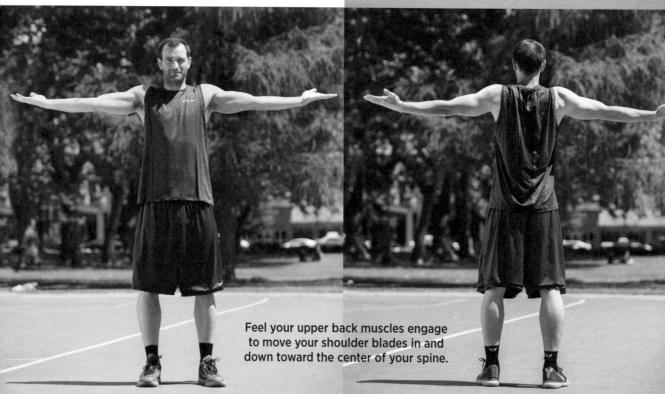

Feel your upper back muscles engage to move your shoulder blades in and down toward the center of your spine.

GAME
PLAN

! My shoulder imbalance is most obvious when:

✓ I'll strike a balance between front body space and back body strength by:

#hitreset

✓ What are you doing to sort out your shoulders today?

KEEP YOUR SHOULDERS FLUID

DO THE
**LITTLE
THINGS**

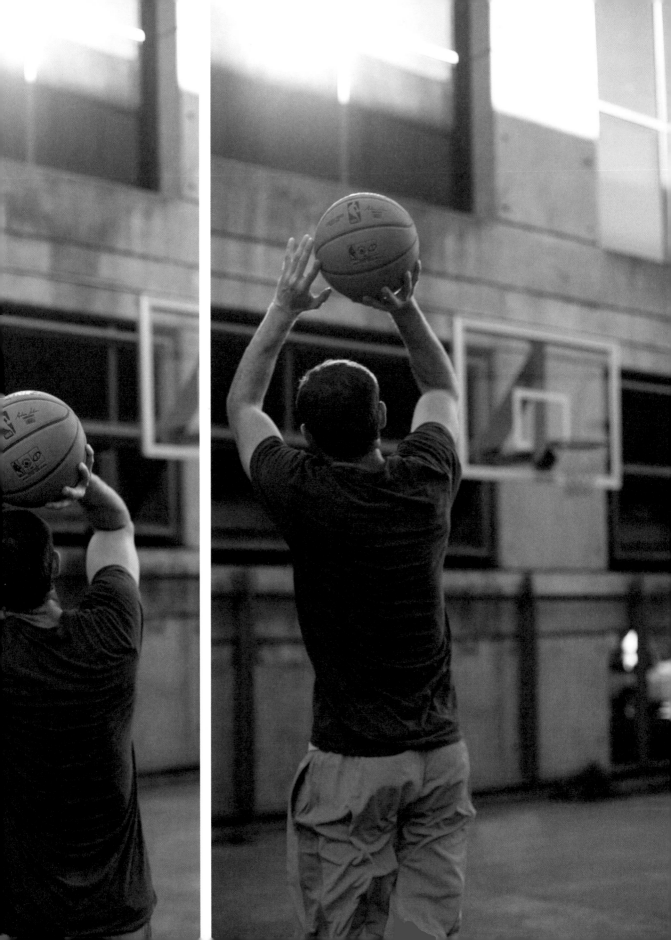

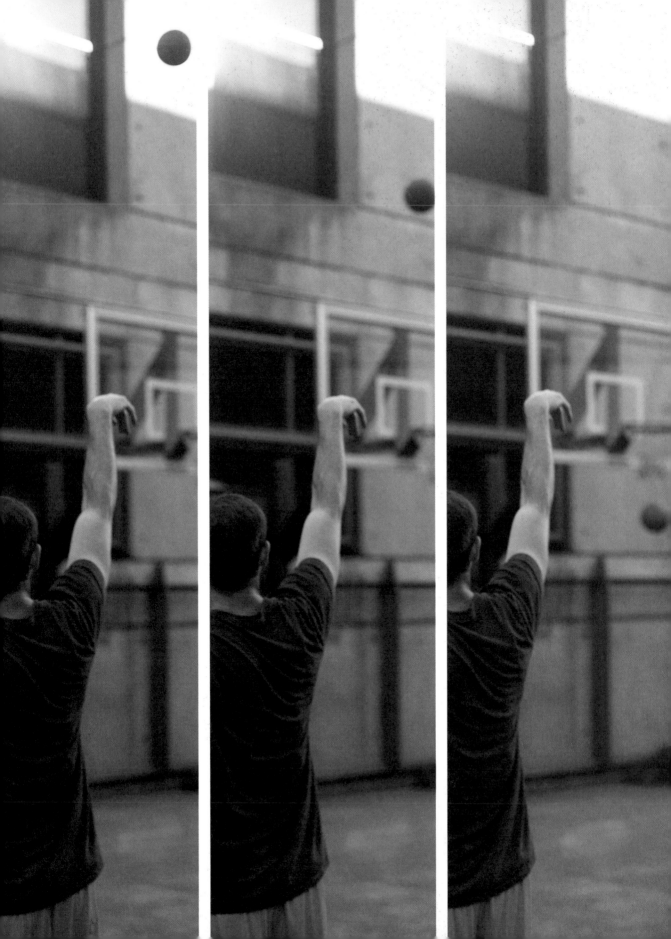

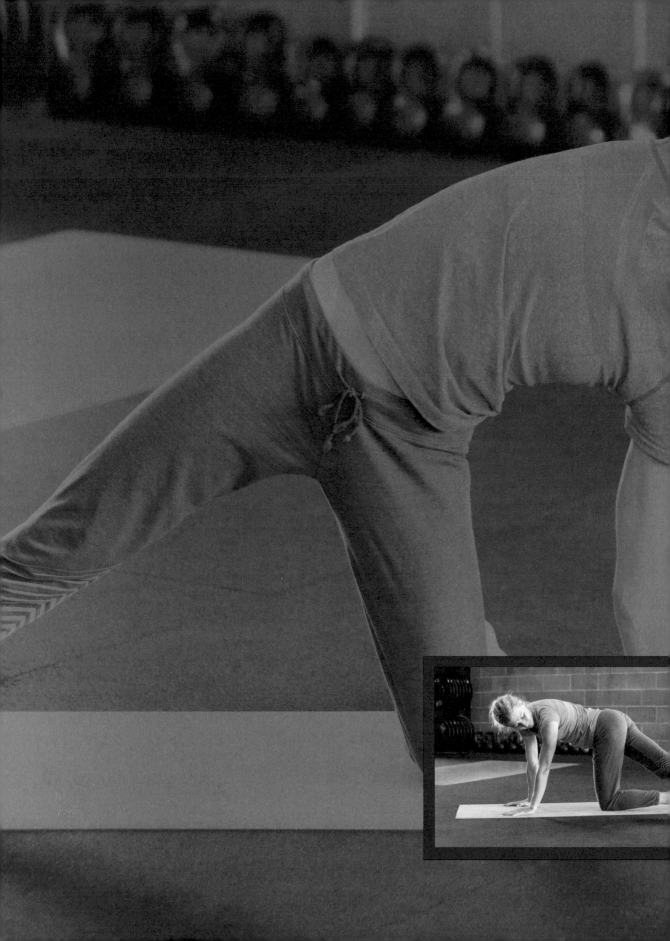

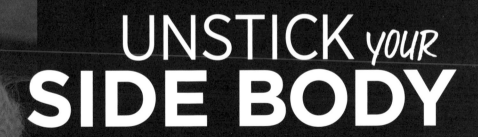

UNSTICK *your* SIDE BODY

While not as contained or specific as areas such as your hips and hamstrings, your side body warrants just as much time and attention. Because we're so forward-oriented in most of our movement, the muscles that live in this region of the body are commonly neglected and as a result become stiff and stuck together.

As you're moving forward—literally and figuratively—toward your goals, it's easy to lose track of what's going on in your side body. Park what initially comes to mind (especially if it involves a muffin top) and consider what's actually happening beneath your skin. There is a group of muscles that are critical for keeping your body stable and upright, and they span an area that extends well beyond your waist.

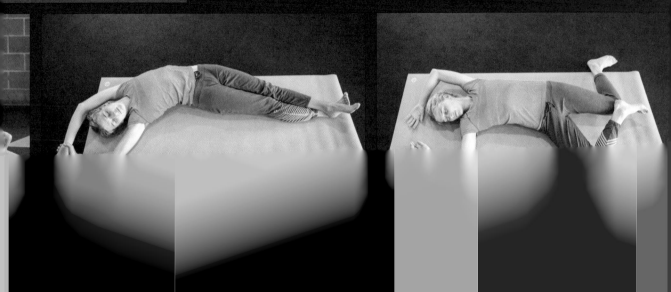

FAQ So what exactly is my side pocket?

Your side pocket includes:

> QL (quadratus lumborum): key back core muscle that lengthens and extends your spine

> external oblique: abdominal muscle that rotates your trunk

> glute max: biggest glute muscle, aka the boss of your push-off

> glute med: key hip stabilizer

> TFL (tensor fasciae latae): hip flexor and stabilizer that assists in turning your thighs in

> psoas/iliacus: the most powerful of your hip flexors, these guys lift your leg forward and assist in turning your thighs out

> vastus lateralis: quad muscle that assists in extending your knee, aka straightens your leg

We've worked most of these areas in previous routines, but now it's time to really lean in. Maintaining side body fluidity will help you feel longer, leaner, and more agile.

! PROBLEM

Stiff, stuck sides lack fluidity

The muscles that live along the sides of your body aren't just stiff, they also get stuck together, kind of like Velcro. This resulting stuckness strains the surrounding areas, limits your range of motion, and increases your injury risk.

✔ SOLUTION

REACH INTO YOUR **SIDE POCKET**

To counter the effects of all your forward action, it's critical that you move outside your usual range of motion daily. For most of us, side bending or any other lateral (side-to-side) movement accomplishes this and increases fluidity through your side body connective tissues to enhance all of your movement.

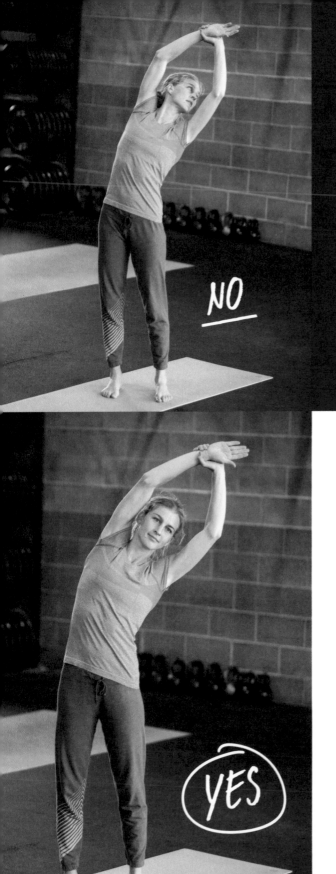

NO

WHERE'S YOUR BEND
COMING FROM?

> Stand in front of a mirror and establish a balanced foundation (p. 61).

> Reach your arms overhead, grab one wrist with your other hand, and bend away from the lifted-arm side.

> Notice where your bend is happening.

  Have your hips shifted more to one side?

  Has your rib cage popped open?

  Are you flopping forward?

YES

✔ CORRECT

> Initiate your bend from your mid-spine (the most mobile point, where movement is supposed to happen)—basically the bottom of your rib cage.

> Don't let anything below your rib cage shift or move—keep your foundation balanced.

> Imagine your body is being pressed between two pieces of glass rather than leaning back or flopping forward.

If back bending is your tendency, you'll need to focus on engaging your obliques to knit your front ribs toward each other.

And if you're forward flopping so that your torso turns toward the floor, you'll need to back off and only bend to the point where you can keep your chest broad and facing forward.

HIT RESET TO UNSTICK YOUR SIDE BODY

ROUTINE

✓ **Reach into Your Side Pocket** (p. 165)

BENEFITS

› Maintain fluidity in the sides of the body

› Counter your habitual forward movement

› Ease muscular imbalances

PRACTICE	Post-workout/recovery
HOW LONG	Hold for 5–8 breaths or 10+ reps/multiple sets for movement
PROPS	Blanket or pillow
RED FLAGS	Spinal compensation via back bending or rounding forward

YOUR BODY IS CAPABLE OF A DYNAMIC RANGE OF MOVEMENT—USE IT ALL!

FAQ How do I stretch my IT bands?

The iliotibial bands (commonly known as the IT bands) are thick bands of connective tissue that live on the sides of your body, extending from your outer hip to outer knee. Their main job is to help stabilize your knees. That's right: Your IT bands are not muscles, so they're not meant to be stretched.

While you might feel discomfort in this area, it's more likely that your surrounding side body muscles need to be addressed because your repetitive forward motion has stiffened your hips and created adhesions—thick misaligned knots of muscle fiber—that place undue stress on the IT bands. If left

unchecked, the problem will ultimately be passed down to your knees per the law of compensation—your body continues transferring stress to the point of least resistance.

What to do? Fear not. While you can't stretch those pesky bands, you can increase circulation through the sides of your body and stretch the tissues around your IT bands. This has an unsticking effect, which will help keep your IT bands happier and better able to do their job of stabilizing your knees, not to mention help keep your body more balanced in general.

REACH INTO YOUR **SIDE POCKET**

RECLINED SIDE BEND

1 Lie down, straighten your legs, and reach your arms overhead.

2 Grab one wrist with your other hand, and bend away from the lifted arm side.

3 Cross your ankles and take your legs in the same direction as the upper body, making an arc from head to toe.

Repeat on your other side.

FLANK

1 Lie on your back and extend your arms open to the sides at shoulder height, palms up.

2 Bring your feet wider than hip width apart and drop your thighs to one side.

3 Put your foot on top of the other thigh, using the weight of that leg to encourage the thigh to rotate farther in the hip joint and drop toward the floor.

4 If it feels too hard to keep your foot on the other leg or if either of your knees are uncomfortable, just rest your foot on the floor instead.

5 Keep both feet flexed.

Repeat on your other side.

Reach forward with the thigh.

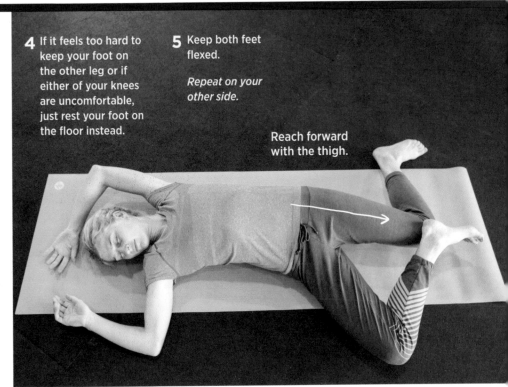

Do this sequence first on one side, then pause and feel the difference before repeating the sequence on the other side.

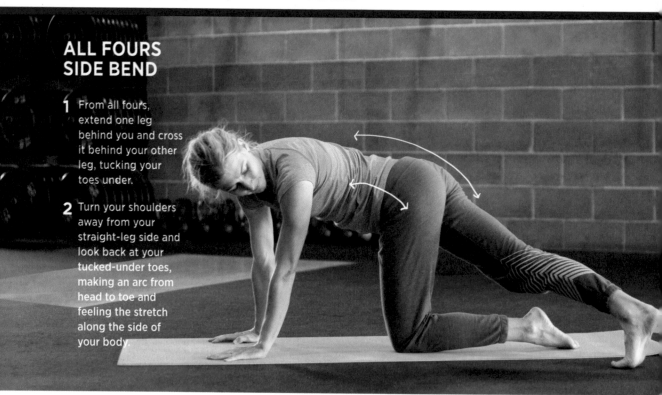

ALL FOURS SIDE BEND

1 From all fours, extend one leg behind you and cross it behind your other leg, tucking your toes under.

2 Turn your shoulders away from your straight-leg side and look back at your tucked-under toes, making an arc from head to toe and feeling the stretch along the side of your body.

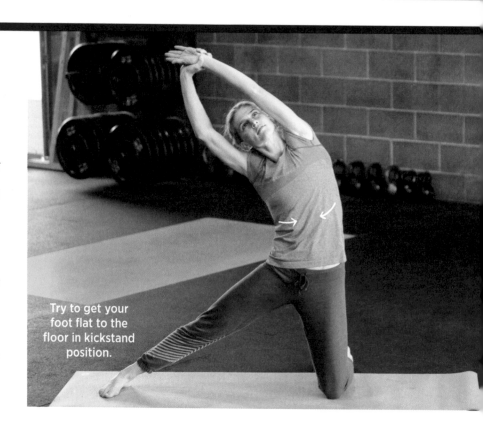

KICKSTAND SIDE BEND

1 From all fours, extend one leg out to the side like a kickstand, lining your foot up with your grounded knee—add padding if needed.

2 Reach your arms overhead, grab your wrist on the opposite side of your body, and bend your torso toward your extended leg.

3 Feel the stretch from your IT band all the way up your torso.

Try to get your foot flat to the floor in kickstand position.

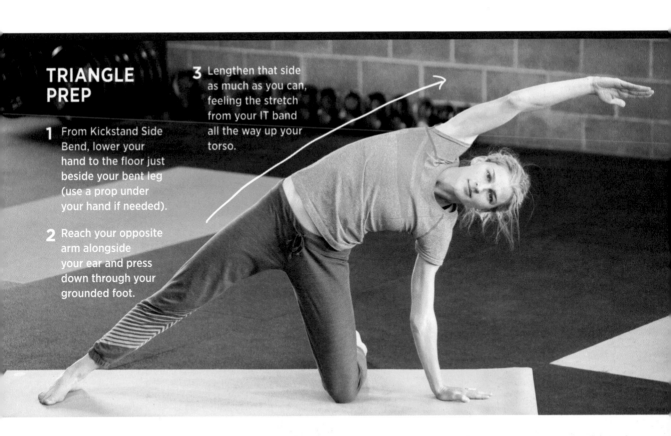

TRIANGLE PREP

1 From Kickstand Side Bend, lower your hand to the floor just beside your bent leg (use a prop under your hand if needed).

2 Reach your opposite arm alongside your ear and press down through your grounded foot.

3 Lengthen that side as much as you can, feeling the stretch from your IT band all the way up your torso.

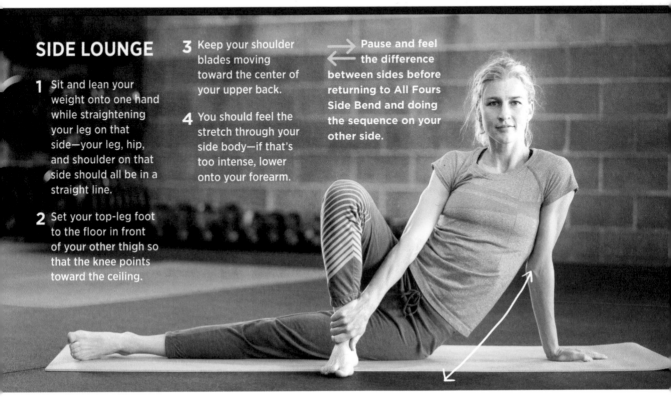

SIDE LOUNGE

1 Sit and lean your weight onto one hand while straightening your leg on that side—your leg, hip, and shoulder on that side should all be in a straight line.

2 Set your top-leg foot to the floor in front of your other thigh so that the knee points toward the ceiling.

3 Keep your shoulder blades moving toward the center of your upper back.

4 You should feel the stretch through your side body—if that's too intense, lower onto your forearm.

Pause and feel the difference between sides before returning to All Fours Side Bend and doing the sequence on your other side.

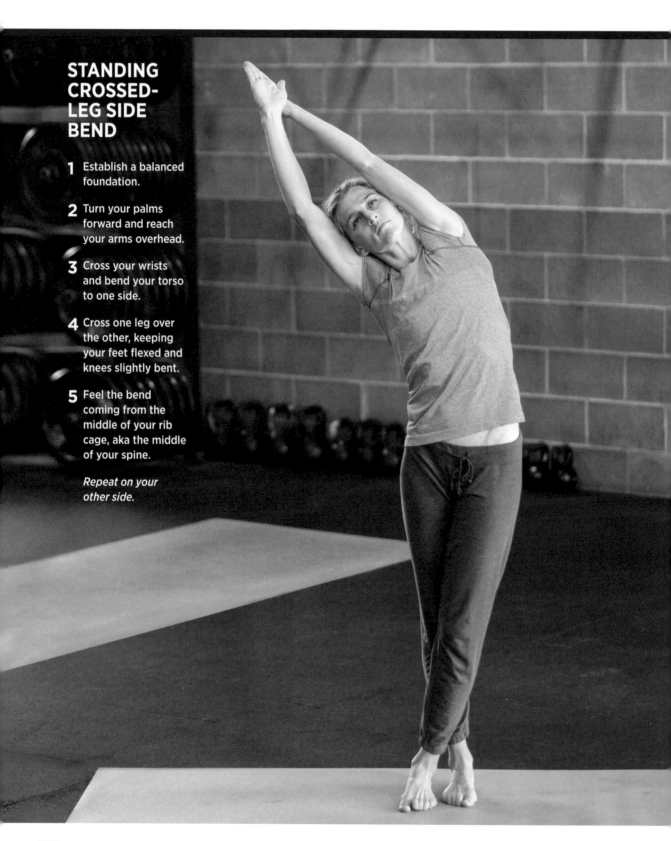

STANDING CROSSED-LEG SIDE BEND

1 Establish a balanced foundation.

2 Turn your palms forward and reach your arms overhead.

3 Cross your wrists and bend your torso to one side.

4 Cross one leg over the other, keeping your feet flexed and knees slightly bent.

5 Feel the bend coming from the middle of your rib cage, aka the middle of your spine.

Repeat on your other side.

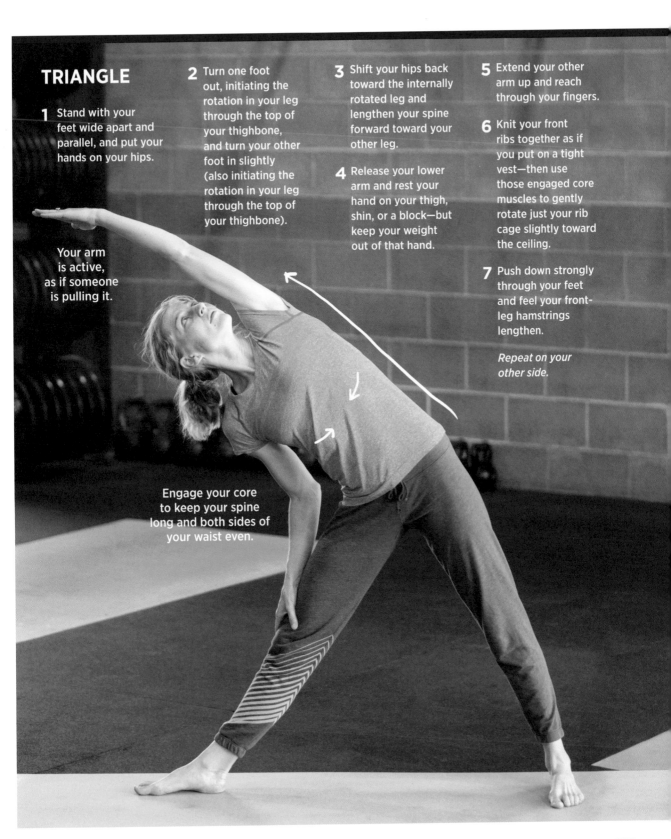

TRIANGLE

1 Stand with your feet wide apart and parallel, and put your hands on your hips.

2 Turn one foot out, initiating the rotation in your leg through the top of your thighbone, and turn your other foot in slightly (also initiating the rotation in your leg through the top of your thighbone).

3 Shift your hips back toward the internally rotated leg and lengthen your spine forward toward your other leg.

4 Release your lower arm and rest your hand on your thigh, shin, or a block—but keep your weight out of that hand.

5 Extend your other arm up and reach through your fingers.

6 Knit your front ribs together as if you put on a tight vest—then use those engaged core muscles to gently rotate just your rib cage slightly toward the ceiling.

7 Push down strongly through your feet and feel your front-leg hamstrings lengthen.

Repeat on your other side.

Your arm is active, as if someone is pulling it.

Engage your core to keep your spine long and both sides of your waist even.

GAME
PLAN

! **Where my sides feel the most stuck, and why:**

✓ **I'll move laterally (side to side) by:**

#hitreset
✓ **What are you doing to unstick your side body today?**

*SIDE BEND
YOUR BOD*

DO THE
**LITTLE
THINGS**

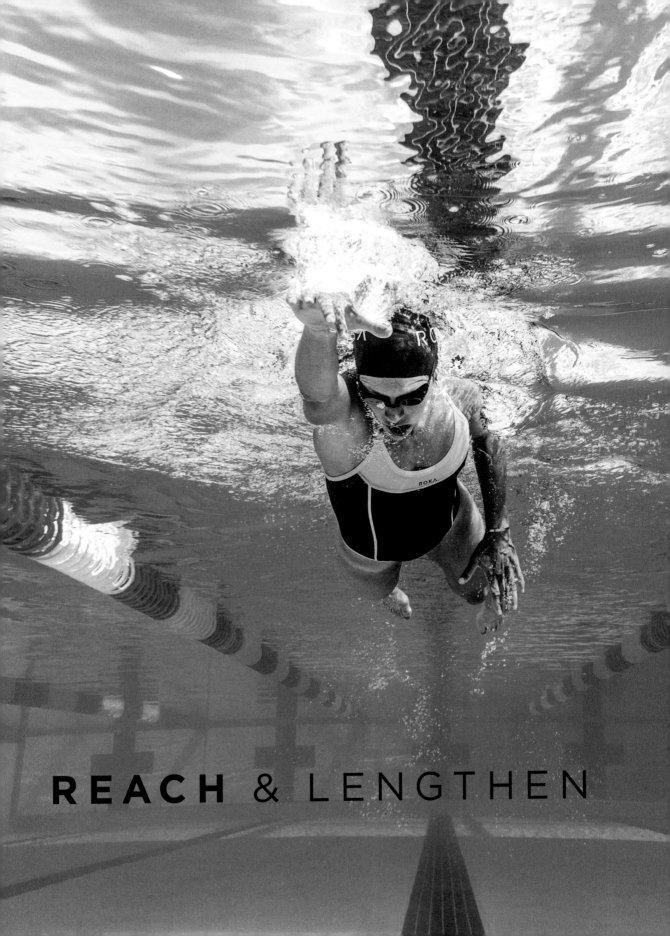

REACH & LENGTHEN

IT'S NOT JUST ABOUT DOING YOGA,
IT'S HOW YOU DO IT

EPILOGUE

MAKE IT HAPPEN

It's not just about doing yoga, it's how you do it. A little bit goes a long way—optimizes your training rather than working against it—*when you're doing the right things*. The self-tests and information in this book have armed you with knowledge about your imbalances and how to fix them. That awareness is step one. Now don't just talk about listening to your body. The next step is to respond—to take action—to systematically address those issues using these solutions.

Stay aware of where you are and, most important, be willing to respond accordingly.

LOVE THE PROCESS

Balance isn't an end goal. It's a way of being—a choice to pay attention to where you are and consciously discern what's needed day to day and moment to moment so that you feel and ultimately perform your best. There will be times when balance feels more or less readily available; embrace the fact that it's always different, which means you'll need to continually assess and fine-tune.

PRE/WARM-UP → **TRAIN/COMPETE** → POST/RECOVER

Each training session or competition is a journey that should have a beginning, middle, and end. Your training and competing is only the middle. Without the beginning (preparation) and the end (recovery) your journey isn't balanced. It's incomplete.

The beginning is your preparation for your workout, whether that's a tempo run or an open-water swim session. This will:

> Activate the muscles that power and support your sport-specific movement

> Bring your mental focus to the task at hand

The end is your recovery, whether you're midweek or on a rest day. This will:

> Ease overworked muscles and address any areas of your body that feel strained

> Consciously correct your body back toward center

Those pre- and post-workout activities optimize your training—and your awareness of balance throughout will help you to continually avoid injuries.

Each day, use the information and tools in this book to create and sustain balance through the journey of each workout. You don't have

	MONDAY	TUESDAY	WEDNESDAY
PRE / WARM-UP	**Feel the Feeling of Achieving Your Goal** *Meditation to ground my goal + set the tone for the week.*	**All Fours Calf Pump** *Calves are sore from yesterday's run so warmed them up!*	**Turn On Your Transverse** **Balance Your Booty** **Strengthen Your Hip Helpers**
WORKOUT	**RUN**	**RUN**	**DAY OFF** *Had more time since not running today. Crosstrained with 3 routines to strengthen my stride.*
POST / RECOVER	**Mitigate Booty Lock** *With extra time on my tighter side (right).*	**Squat Calf Pump** *Still feeling stiff so hit them with a more aggressive stretch while still warm.*	

to do everything in a week or do an entire routine to make an impact. Think about what you're doing and why. Aim to do a little bit every day—even if it's just one pose—knowing that anything is better than nothing and that consistency is key.

Remember that your body wants balance and so it will respond to even the subtlest reminders you give and the smallest efforts you make to reestablish a sense of center. When you experience the difference this approach to yoga makes, consistent practice will feel like a priority and an integrated part of your lifestyle rather than another thing on your to-do list.

In addition, revisit the self-tests and techniques periodically, knowing that you'll respond differently depending on where you are in your season or training cycle. Think of each area of your body as a connected system, and over time as you work through these Resets, you'll deepen your knowledge of how each area of the body works and, ultimately, how they all function together to work optimally as the integrated unit your body is engineered to be.

Practice serves as a potent reminder of where you are and what you're working toward.

SUSTAIN BALANCE AND WIN

THURSDAY	FRIDAY	SATURDAY	SUNDAY
Matching Breath	**Back Core Isolation Flow**	**Forward Fold with bend & stretch**	
Stressful day at work so focused on breath while getting ready to go run.	*Wanted to get some functional core in so used this as a warm-up … tough!*	*Overslept so not much time, but needed a wake-up.*	
RUN	**RUN**	**LONG RUN**	**REST DAY**
Reclined Windshield Wipers	**Wall Chest Stretch**	**Restore Your Range**	**Establish a Blueprint for Center**
Sore hips but didn't feel like stretching, so this is better than nothing.	*Posture feels really rounded after a lot of desk time. More noticeable on today's run so hit up the best chest stretch.*	*Hams super sore, no gas left for active stretching.*	*To help reestablish center + aid recovery.*

ROUTINES

PRE-WORKOUT OR CROSSTRAINING

Hold for 5–8 breaths
or 10+ reps/multiple sets
for movement

>> Breathe & Focus routines (pp. 24–29)
can be done anytime.

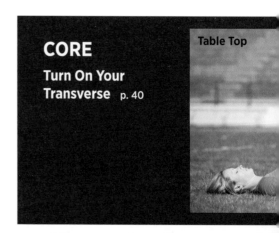

CORE

Turn On Your Transverse p. 40

Table Top

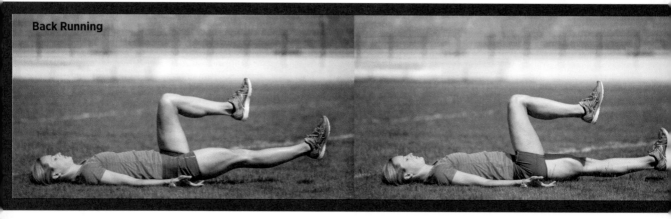

Back Running

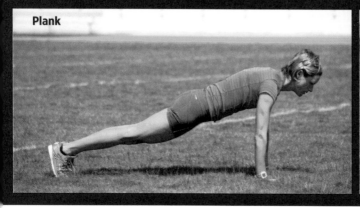

Plank

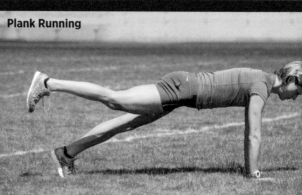

Plank Running

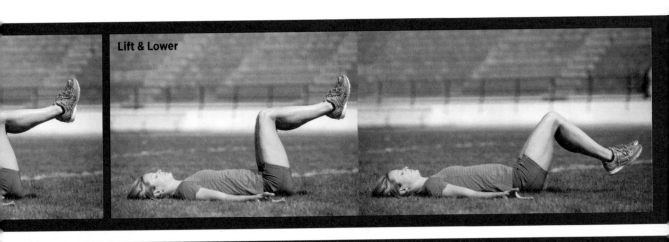

Lift & Lower

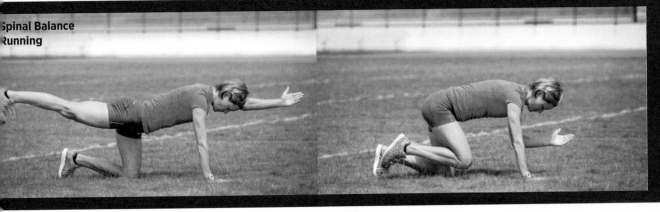

**Spinal Balance
Running**

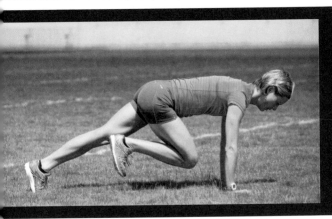

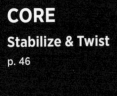

CORE
Stabilize & Twist
p. 46

**Seated
Twisting**

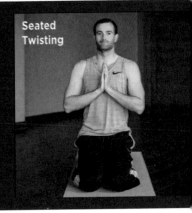

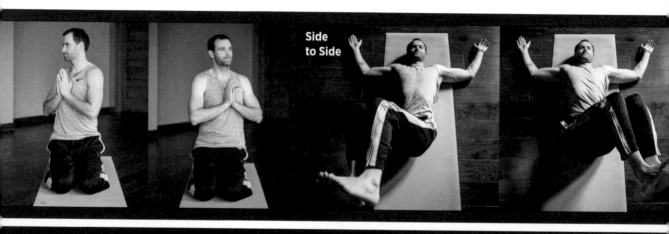

Side to Side

CORE

Find Your Back Pack p. 50

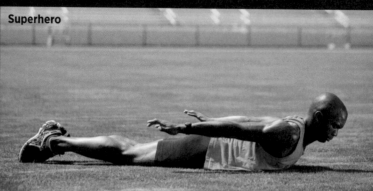

Superhero

Back Core Isolation

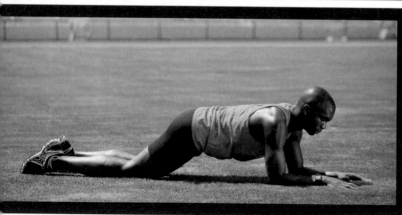

Boat

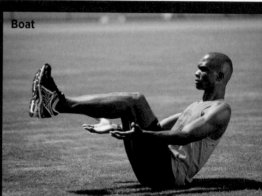

FOUNDATION

Fix Your Feet
p. 63

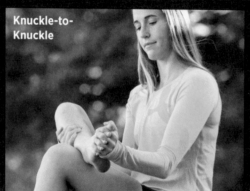

Knuckle-to-Knuckle

Toe Yoga

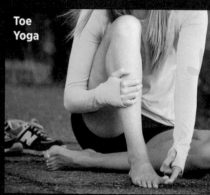

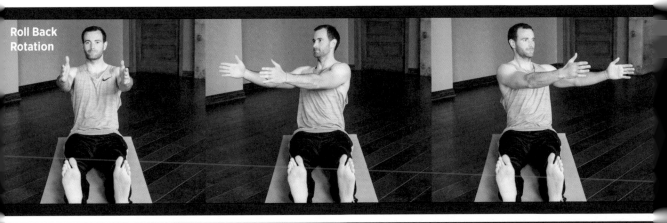
Roll Back Rotation

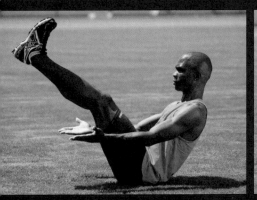
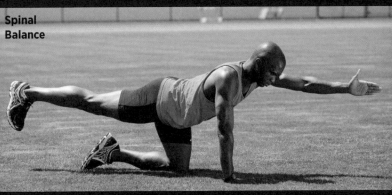
Back Core Isolation Flow

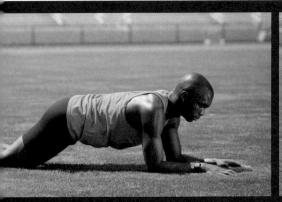
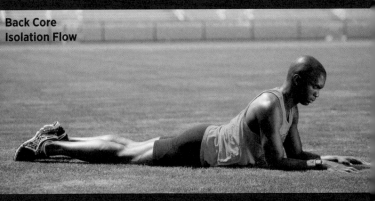
Spinal Balance

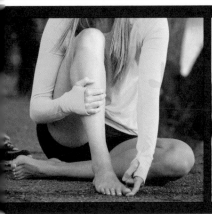
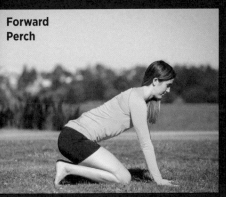
Forward Perch

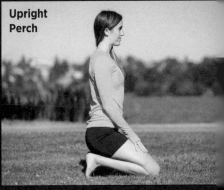
Upright Perch

FOUNDATION

Pump Your Calves
p. 66

**Hammy Time
Point & Flex**

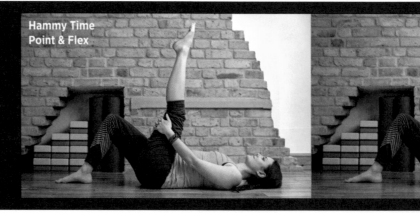

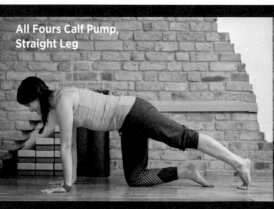

**All Fours Calf Pump,
Straight Leg**

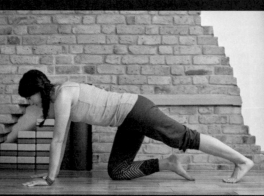

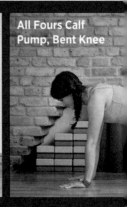

**All Fours Calf
Pump, Bent Knee**

KNEES

Align Your Stride
p. 79

**Low
Lunge**

⇄

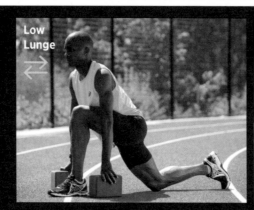

Runner's Lunge

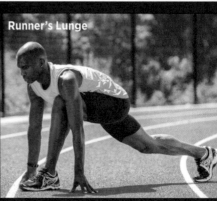

**Lunge
Flow**

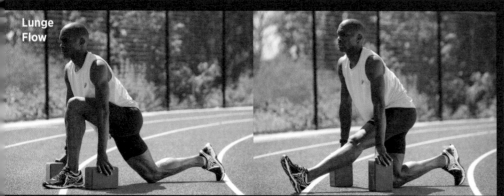

Lizard

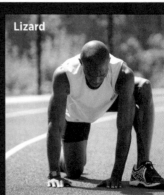

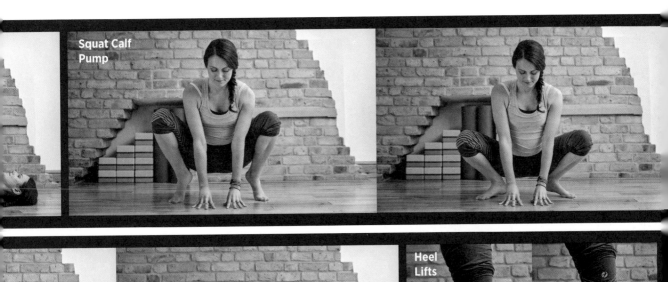

Squat Calf Pump

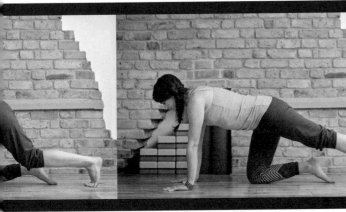

Heel Lifts

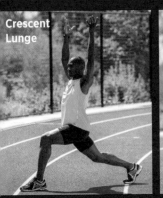

Crescent Lunge

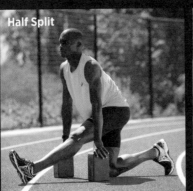

Half Split

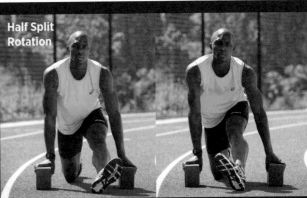

Half Split Rotation

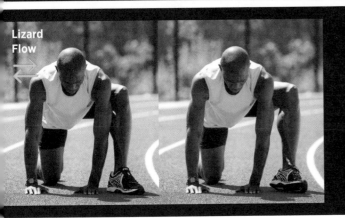

Lizard Flow

HAMSTRINGS

Find Fluidity p. 92

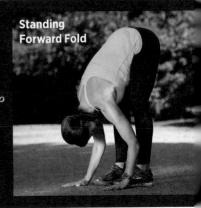

Standing Forward Fold

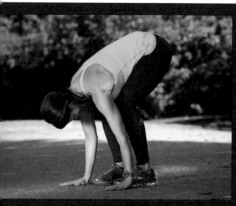

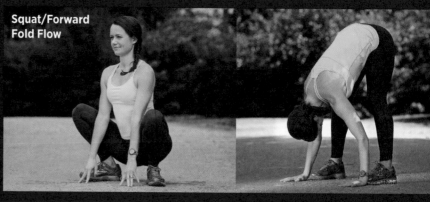

Squat/Forward Fold Flow

BUTT

Balance Your Booty p. 111

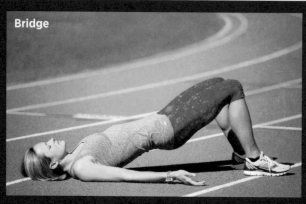

Bridge

Bridge Flow

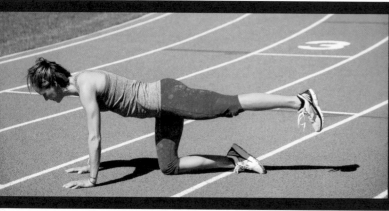

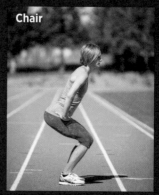

Chair

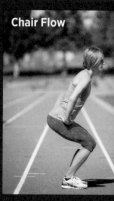

Chair Flow

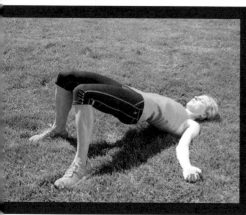

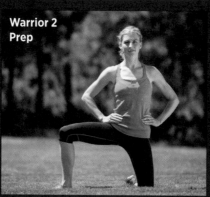

Warrior 2 Prep

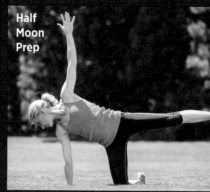

Half Moon Prep

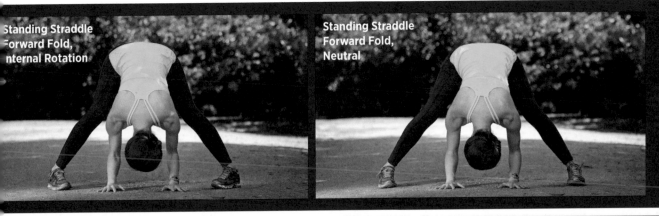

Standing Straddle Forward Fold, Internal Rotation

Standing Straddle Forward Fold, Neutral

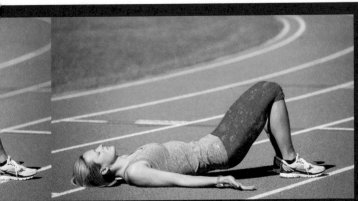

All Fours Running

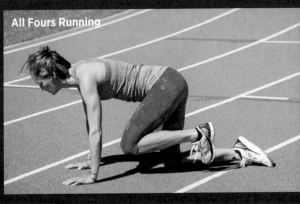

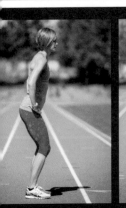

Single-Leg Balance

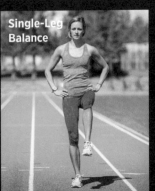

HIPS

Strengthen Your Hip Helpers p. 132

Wide Bridge Flow

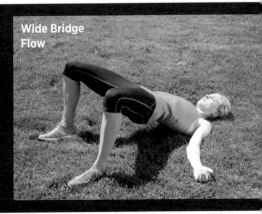

Horse

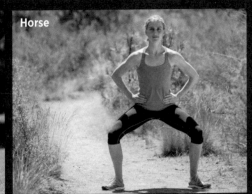

Warrior 2

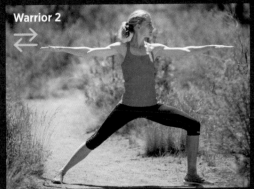

Tree Prep

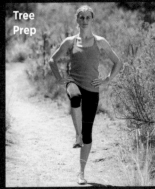

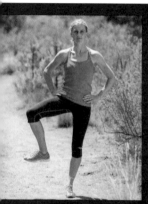

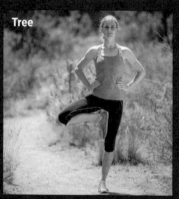
Tree

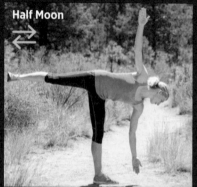
Half Moon

SHOULDERS
Find Your Back Pack p. 50 +
BONUS POSE p. 156

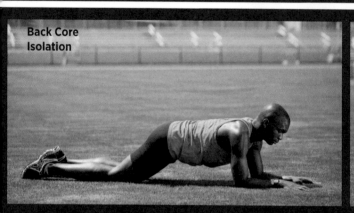
Back Core Isolation

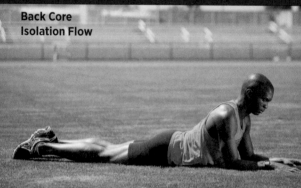
Back Core Isolation Flow

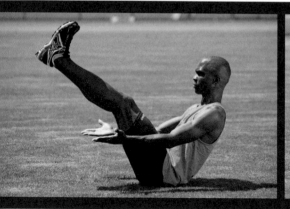

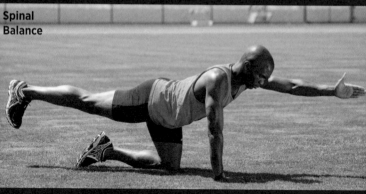
Spinal Balance

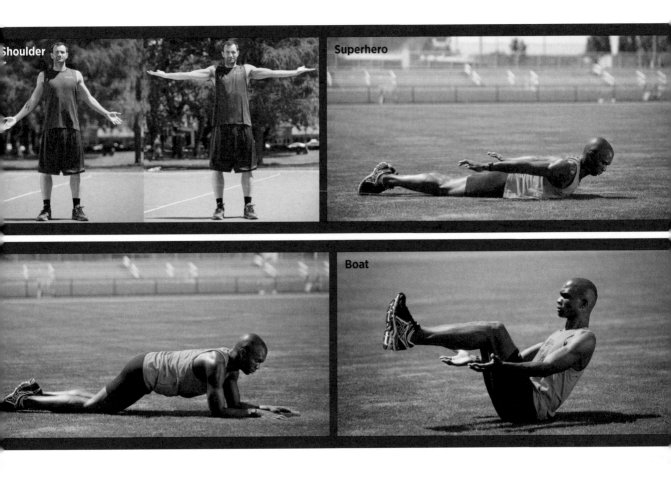

Shoulder

Superhero

Boat

DO A LITTLE BIT EVERY DAY

POST-WORKOUT OR RECOVERY DAYS

Hold for 5–8 breaths or 10+ reps/multiple sets for movement

BALANCE
Establish a Blueprint for Center p. 9

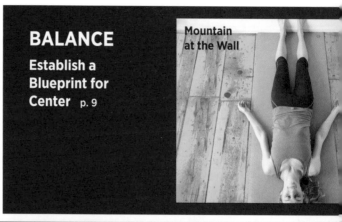

Mountain at the Wall

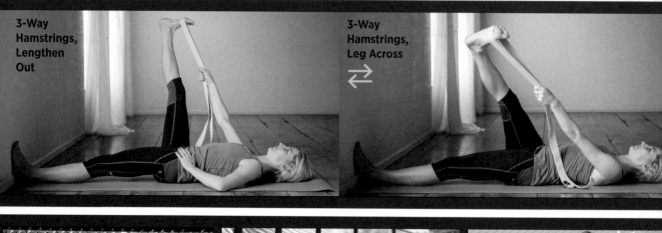

3-Way Hamstrings, Lengthen Out

3-Way Hamstrings, Leg Across

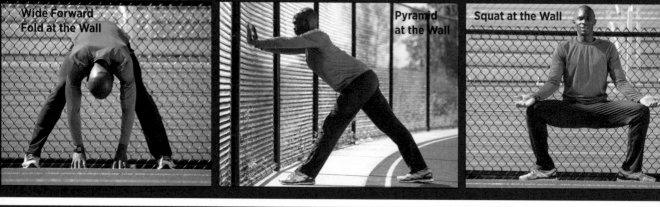

Wide Forward Fold at the Wall

Pyramid at the Wall

Squat at the Wall

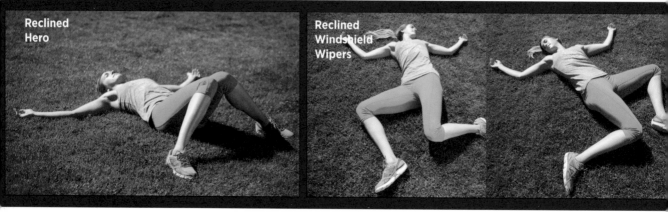

Reclined Hero

Reclined Windshield Wipers

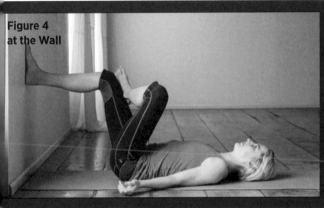

Figure 4
at the Wall

3-Way
Hamstrings,
Lengthen Up
⇄

HAMSTRINGS

**Restore Your
Range** p. 98

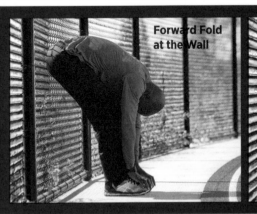

Forward Fold
at the Wall

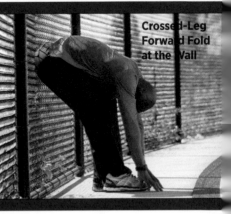

Crossed-Leg
Forward Fold
at the Wall

HIPS

**Mitigate Booty
Lock** p. 123

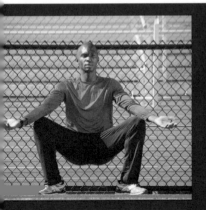

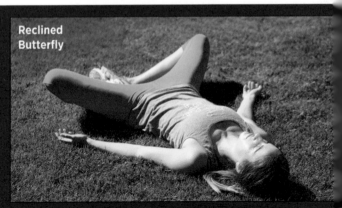

Reclined
Butterfly

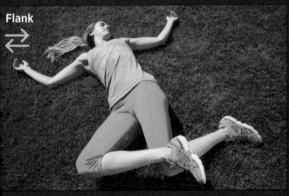

Flank
⇄

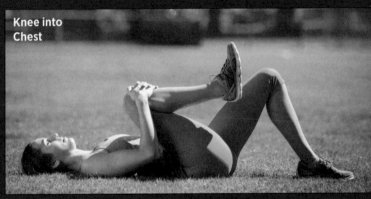

Knee into
Chest

Half Happy Baby

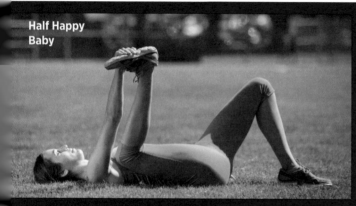

Figure 4

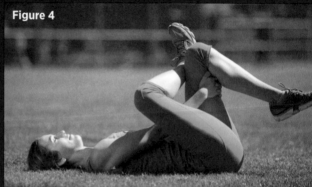

SHOULDERS

Stretch Your Chest
p. 150

Shoulder Circles

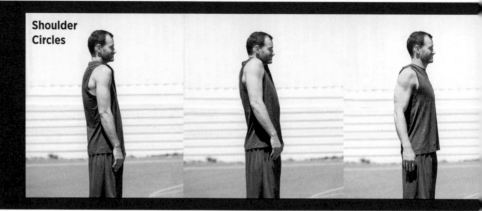

Wall Chest Stretch

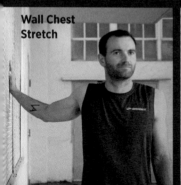

Half Dragonfly at the Wall

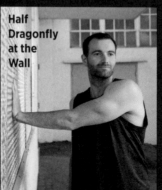

Shower

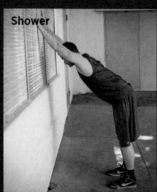

SIDE BODY

Reach into Your Side Pocket p. 165

All Fours Side Bend
⇄

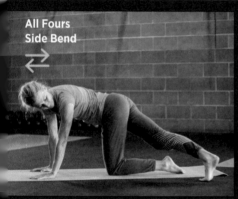

Triangle Prep

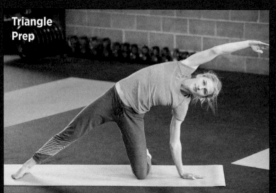

Kickstand Side Bend

Reclined Shoelace
⇄

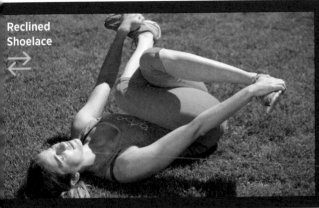

Happy Baby

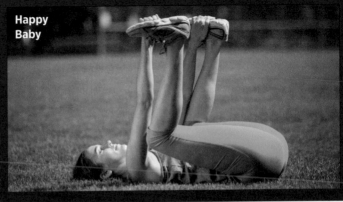

Chest Expansion

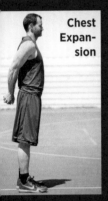

Moving Goalpost

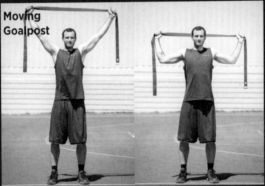

Rotator Cuff Stretch

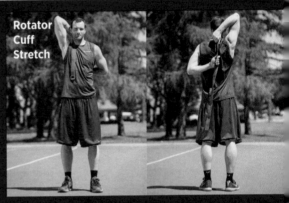

Reclined Side Bend

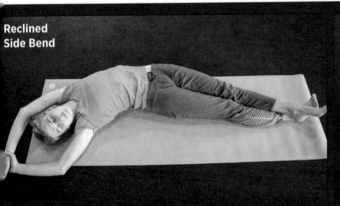

Flank

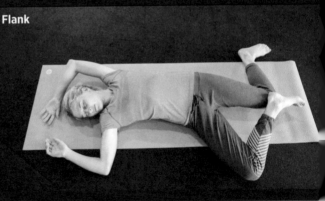

Side Lounge
⇄

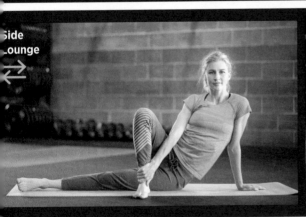

Standing Crossed-Leg Side Bend

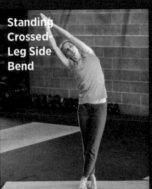

Triangle

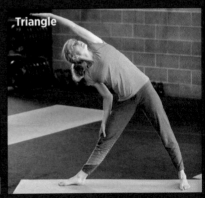

GLOSSARY

ACTIVE STRETCHING
Dynamic stretches that increase blood flow while lengthening the tissue and that allow you to increase the intensity on your own. These poses are most effective pre-workout, although they can be done post-workout as well.

BIOMECHANICS
The way all your parts—including your bones, connective tissue, and muscles—are engineered to work together.

BOOTY LOCK
Just what it sounds like: super-sore butt and limited hip mobility resulting from tight hips and glutes.

COMPENSATION
The body's intrinsic and subconscious effort to find balance in the presence of compensation.

EXTERNAL ROTATION
Aka turn out—think rotating your legs so your toes point out or rotating your arms so your palms face forward.

FASCIA/DEEP FASCIA
The fabric that holds our cells together. Deep fascia specifically holds our muscle cells together and organizes them into specific muscle bellies.

FAST-TWITCH MUSCLES
Muscles that provide explosive power—think sprinters and jumpers.

ADHESION Muscles have tons of fibers that are held in place by layers of deep fascia. Those are meant to align and slide over each other. When our fascia get cranky, thick, misaligned knots can form and cause an array of issues.

ATHLETE Anyone who values an active, healthy lifestyle and/or has made a conscious decision to pursue a sports or fitness goal.

BALANCE Equilibrium.

CONNECTIVE TISSUE Sheets of fascia, ligaments, membranes, blood vessels, and more that connects stuff in your body.

EASEFUL Minimal stress and maximum effectiveness.

ECCENTRIC STRENGTH When tissues contract while they're lengthening.

FLEXIBILITY The ability to access the full range of motion of any joint.

FLUIDITY Being able to move with optimal power and minimal dysfunction. This brings a feeling of freedom!

FUNCTIONAL Practical.

INTERNAL ROTATION
Aka turn in—think rotating your legs so that your toes point in (pigeon-toed) or rotating your arms so that your palms face back.

INTRINSIC MUSCLES
The little guys that provide stability, kind of like little helpers that provide support to align joints so your power muscles can create movement safely and effectively.

THE LAW OF COMPENSATION
When movement meets restriction and force continues to be applied, that force will transfer to the next available point of least resistance.

RANGE OF MOTION
The movement available in a particular joint.

SLOW-TWITCH MUSCLES Muscles that provide stability and endurance—think distance runners.

SPRAIN A stretch or tear in a ligament.

MUSCLE BELLY
The meat!

PASSIVE STRETCHING More restorative stretches that rely on external forces such as gravity or props to ease the muscles that have worked hard for you by softening their surrounding connective tissues. It's important to focus on these guys post-workout.

PULLED MUSCLE
See strain/strained muscle.

STRAIN/STRAINED MUSCLE Stressing the muscle to the point of tearing the tissue.

TENSION Patterned, inefficient use of energy.

RESET

A yoga solution that eases imbalance.

ACKNOWLEDGMENTS

Namaste is one of the few Sanskrit words I use when I teach. From the ancient language of yoga, it translates to "the light in me honors the light in you," kind of like a yogic fist bump.

After I'd been teaching for several years, my dad, who regularly attended my classes, asked me, "Why do you always say, 'Have a nice day,' at the end of class?" "Have a nice day," I repeated aloud, laughing. I could see how my dad thought I had been saying that, rather than *namaste*. This still brings a smile to my face. I have to thank my dad for reminding me to convey my message in language my audience can truly understand. Now, as I reflect on the years that this book has been in the making, I send a big yogic fist bump—thank you—to the many people without whose support and guidance this book would not exist:

To my mom, the first person to encourage me to follow my heart and pursue my passion for yoga. Thank you for helping me find my way as an athlete.

To my other half, my husband, Mark. Thank you for encouraging me to dream big and for helping me connect the dots to manifest my goals. And for supporting me in redefining and settling into balance daily.

To my daughter, Rose, who was in my belly during the production of this book. Thank you for choosing me to be your mama and for teaching me that mothering you is the ultimate meditation.

To my colleagues, Team Jasyoga. Thank you for waving the Reset Revolution flag like bosses.

To all my teachers. Thank you, Richelle Ricard, The Yoga Engineer, for keeping me grounded in functional anatomy.

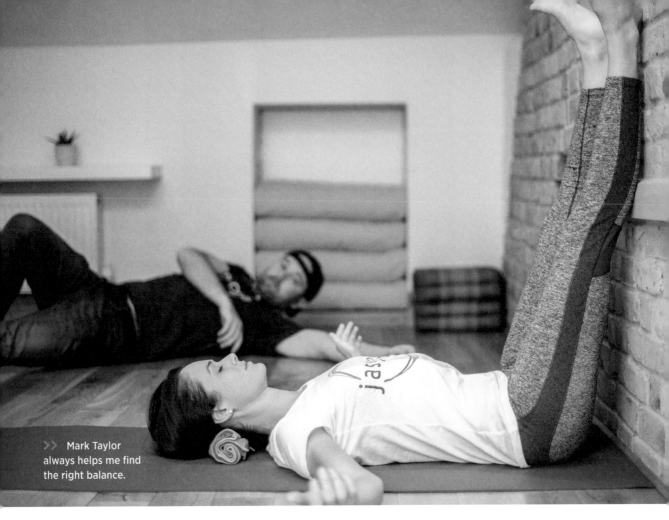

>> Mark Taylor always helps me find the right balance.

To the athletes featured in the pages of this book. Lauren, you are my hero. Linsey, Norris, Casey, and Brianna, I am your biggest admirer. Thank you all for your belief and collaboration.

To my apparel sponsor and all the women of Oiselle. Thank you for inspiring me to woman up and stretch my wingspan, and for all the #flystyle.

To my editor, Renee Jardine, and VeloPress. Thank you for believing in the potential of this book to change the game.

To photographers Claire Pepper, Justin Bailie, Hilary Dahl, and James Finlay. Thank you for your artistry and hearts on these pages.

And most important, to you, the athletes of the Reset Revolution. You are my muse and I hope that every day you use these practices to help you feel more balanced and easeful— and that every time you step on the mat, you lessen the gap between where you are now and where you want to be.

Namaste.

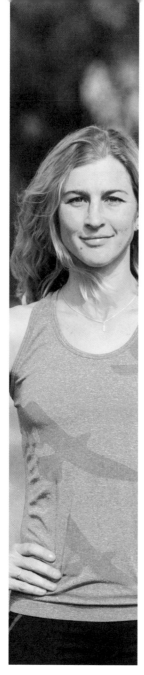
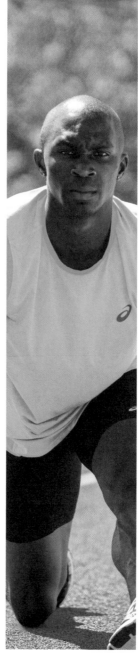
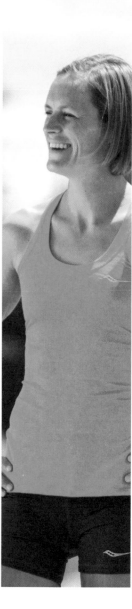

ABOUT THE
ATHLETES
Throughout this book, real athletes lead you back into balance.

Lauren Fleshman
Aka Fleshman Flyer, Lauren is a pro runner with Oiselle, five-time NCAA champ, two-time U.S. champ, cofounder of Picky Bars, and author of *Believe Training Journal*. She loves side bending.
www.asklaurenfleshman.com

Norris Frederick
As an elite long jumper, Norris can literally fly.
www.norrisfrederick.com

Linsey Corbin
Linsey is a pro triathlete, five-time Ironman champ, and American record holder. She also planks like a boss.
www.linseycorbin.com

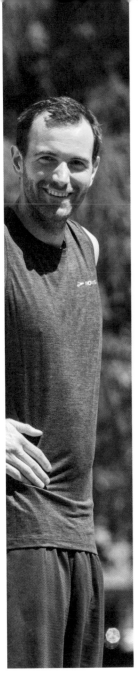

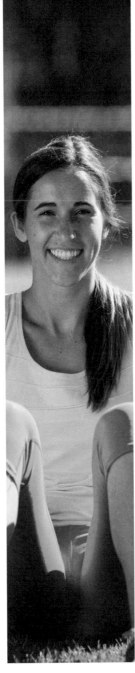

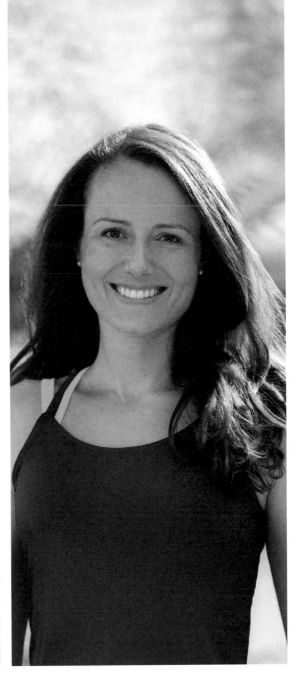

Casey Pursell

Casey is a former collegiate basketball player who has used yoga to help recover from knee injuries and continues to Hit Reset regularly to keep his gun show in check.

Brianna Sweeney

A former collegiate soccer player, Brianna is a Jasyoga coach and world traveler whom you can count on to encourage you to "treat yo-self" with post-Reset donuts or beer.

Erin Taylor

A former collegiate basketball player and the leader of the Reset Revolution, Erin helps athletes use yoga to change the game. She loves a good run—you'll always find her with her legs up the wall afterward.
www.jasyoga.com

ABOUT THE
AUTHOR

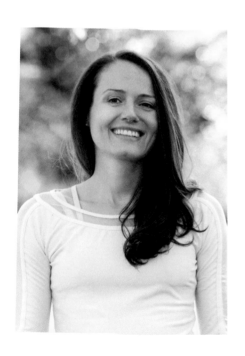

Erin Taylor is an international leader in yoga for athletes. It was her own experience of being sidelined by injury as a collegiate basketball player that first showed her how yoga can be the Reset that brings athletes back into balance.

Erin founded Jasyoga with the goal of providing practical yoga solutions to as many people as possible. Jasyoga equips athletes with powerful skills to prevent injuries and enhance recovery, optimizing performance in sport and life. With operations in the Unites States and the United Kingdom, Jasyoga coaches abandon the traditional studio setting and meet athletes wherever they work out. Over the last decade, Erin has infused meditation, functional anatomy, and physical therapy techniques into her practice. Now accessible anytime, anywhere via her online video platform, Erin's approach has been widely embraced by athletes ranging from recreational to elite over the last decade, and can be configured to help anyone achieve their goals.

Erin is a regular contributor to popular health and fitness blogs and publications. In addition to privately coaching sports teams and athletes, she hosts popular teacher trainings and yoga-for-athlete certification programs. She lives in London with her husband and daughter.

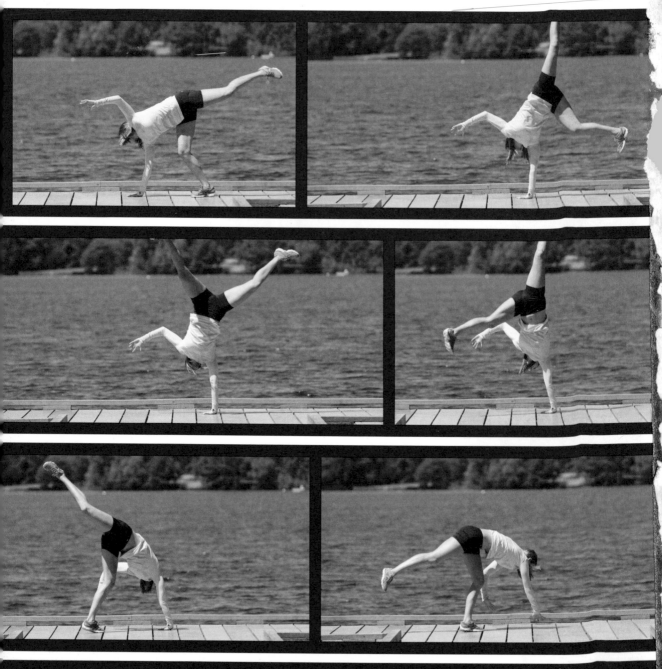

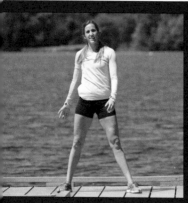

BALANCING STRENGTH
& FLEXIBILITY
BRINGS **FREEDOM**.
GET AFTER IT!